ADVANCES IN
Family Practice Nursing

Editor-in-Chief
Geri C. Reeves, PhD, APRN, FNP-BC

Associate Editors
Sharon L. Holley, DNP, CNM, FACNM

Linda J. Keilman, DNP, GNP-BC, FAANP

Imelda Reyes, DNP, MPH, APRN, CPNP-PC, FNP-BC, FAANP

ELSEVIER

PHILADELPHIA   LONDON   TORONTO   MONTREAL   SYDNEY   TOKYO

Editor: Kerry Holland
Developmental Editor: Casey Potter

Editorial Office:
Elsevier
1600 John F. Kennedy Blvd,
Suite 1800
Philadelphia, PA 19103-2899

International Standard Serial Number: 2589-4722
International Standard Book Number: 978-0-323-65368-8

ADVANCES IN
Family Practice Nursing

Editor-in-Chief

GERI C. REEVES, PhD, APRN, FNP-BC, Assistant Professor, Vanderbilt University School of Nursing, Nashville, Tennessee

Associate Editors

SHARON L. HOLLEY, DNP, CNM, FACNM, Chief, Division of Midwifery & Community Health, Associate Professor, Department of OB-Gyn at University of Massachusetts Medical School-Baystate, Baystate Medical Center, Springfield, Massachusetts

LINDA J. KEILMAN, DNP, GNP-BC, FAANP, Associate Professor, Director AGPCNP Program, Gerontological Nurse Practitioner, Michigan State University, College of Nursing, East Lansing, Michigan

IMELDA REYES, DNP, MPH, APRN, CPNP-PC, FNP-BC, FAANP, Associate Clinical Professor, Pediatric Primary Care NP Specialty Coordinator, DNP Population Health Track Coordinator, Emory University, Nell Hodgson Woodruff School of Nursing, Atlanta, Georgia

CONTRIBUTORS

NATALIE R. BAKER, DNP, ANP-BC, GNP-BC, GS-C, FAANP, Associate Professor, The University of Alabama at Birmingham School of Nursing, Birmingham, Alabama, USA

AMY BLUMLING, RN, CPNP-PC, Nell Hodgson Woodruff School of Nursing, Atlanta, Georgia, USA

SUSAN BRASHER, PhD, MS, CPNP-PC, Nell Hodgson Woodruff School of Nursing, Atlanta, Georgia, USA

SHARRON CLOSE, PhD, MS, CPNP-PC, FAAN, Nell Hodgson Woodruff School of Nursing, Department of Human Genetics, eXtraordinarY Clinic, Emory School of Medicine, Atlanta, Georgia, USA

KATHLEEN DANHAUSEN, MSN, MPH, CNM, Instructor of Clinical Nursing, Vanderbilt University School of Nursing, Nashville, Tennessee, USA

NICOLE V. DAVIS, MSN, FNP, Family Nurse Practitioner, Unity Health Care, Washington, DC, USA

KATHERINE DONTJE, PhD, FNP-BC, FAANP, Associate Professor, College of Nursing, Michigan State University, East Lansing, Michigan, USA

DANIELLE G. DOOLEY, MD, MPhil, Assistant Professor of Pediatrics, George Washington University School of Medicine and Health Sciences, Child Health Advocacy Institute, Children's National Health System, Washington, DC, USA

DEBORAH DUNN, EdD, MSN, GNP-BC, ACNS-BC, GS-C, Dean, The Graduate School, Director, Center for Research, Professor of Nursing, Madonna University, Livonia, Michigan, USA

OLANREWAJU O. FALUSI, MD, Assistant Professor of Pediatrics, George Washington University School of Medicine and Health Sciences, Child Health Advocacy Institute, Children's National Health System, Washington, DC, USA

CYNTHIA GERSTENLAUER, ANP-BC, GCNS-BC, CDE, CCD, Nurse Practitioner, Troy Internal Medicine, Troy, Michigan, USA

DONNA JACKSON-KÖHLIN, CNM, MSN, CCHP, Baystate Midwifery and Women's Health Clinician, Baystate Midwifery Education Program, Faculty Educator, Baystate Health Systems, Springfield, Massachusetts, USA

KIMBERLY R. JOO, DNP, APRN-CNP, CNE, EBP-C, Assistant Professor of Clinical Practice, The Ohio State University, College of Nursing, Columbus, Ohio, USA; Nurse Practitioner, Dayton Children's Hospital, Springboro Urgent Care, Kids Express, Dayton, Ohio, USA

DAVID KATTAN, MD, MPH, Section Head of Family Planning, Assistant Professor, Department of Obstetrics and Gynecology, University of Massachusetts Medical School-Baystate, Springfield, Massachusetts, USA

LINDA J. KEILMAN, DNP, GNP-BC, FAANP, Associate Professor, Director AGPCNP Program, Gerontological Nurse Practitioner, Michigan State University, College of Nursing, East Lansing, Michigan, USA

JENNIFER KIM, DNP, GNP-BC, GS-C, FNAP, FAANP, Assistant Professor, Vanderbilt University School of Nursing, Nashville, Tennessee, USA

TERESA KIRESUK, DNP, APRN, AGPCNP-C, Director, Adult Gerontology Primary Care Nurse Practitioner Online Program, Associate Professor, College of Nursing and Public Health, South University, Savannah, Georgia, USA

ASHLEY DARCY MAHONEY, PhD, NNP-BC, FAAN, Associate Professor, Neonatal Nurse Practitioner, The George Washington University School of Nursing, Director of Infant Research GWU Autism and Neurodevelopmental Disorders Institute, Neonatal Nurse Practitioner, Mednax-South Dade Neonatology, Washington, DC, USA

KRISTY MARTYN, PhD, CPNP-PC, FAAN, Nell Hodgson Woodruff School of Nursing, Atlanta, Georgia, USA

ELIZABETH MUNOZ, CNM, MSN, Vanderbilt University School of Nursing, Nashville, Tennessee, USA

DOUGLAS P. OLSEN, PhD, RN, Associate Professor, Michigan State University, College of Nursing, East Lansing, Michigan, USA; Sechnov University, Moscow, Russia

GEORGE BYRON PERAZA-SMITH, DNP, APRN, GNP-BC, GS-C, CNE, FAANP, Program Director, DNP and Associate Professor, College of Nursing and Public Health, South University, Savannah, Georgia, USA

NEENA QASBA, MD, MPH, Assistant Professor, Department of Obstetrics and Gynecology, University of Massachusetts Medical School-Baystate, Baystate Medical Center, Springfield, Massachusetts, USA

IMELDA REYES, DNP, MPH, RN, CPNP-PC, FNP-BC, FAANP, Associate Clinical Professor, Pediatric Primary Care NP Specialty Coordinator, DNP Population Health Track Coordinator, Emory University, Nell Hodgson Woodruff School of Nursing, Atlanta, Georgia, USA

TANEESHA REYNOLDS, MSN, MBA, CNM, Instructor of Clinical Nursing, Vanderbilt University School of Nursing, Nashville, Tennessee, USA

HEATHER ROBBINS, DNP, MBA, RN, Vanderbilt University School of Nursing, Nashville, Tennessee, USA

JEANNIE RODRIGUEZ, PhD, RN, CPNP-PC, Research Assistant Professor, Pediatrics, Emory University, Nell Hodgson Woodruff School of Nursing, Atlanta, Georgia, USA

MICHELLE STEPHENS, PhD, MSN, PNP, University of California, San Francisco, School of Nursing, Department of Family Health Care Nursing, San Francisco, California, USA

AMY TALBOY, MD, Department of Human Genetics, eXtraordinarY Clinic, Emory School of Medicine, Atlanta, Georgia, USA

SUSAN G. WIERS, DNP, FNP-BC, Assistant Professor - Clinical, Wayne State University, Detroit, Michigan, USA

ADVANCES IN
Family Practice Nursing

CONTENTS   VOLUME 1 • 2019

Adult/Geriatric

Individualized Approach to Hypertension Management Through Shared Decision Making
Katherine Dontje

Best Practices in the Management of Major Depression for Older Adults in Primary Care
George Byron Peraza-Smith and Teresa Kiresuk

Travel Health for Older Adults
Cynthia Gerstenlauer

Ethical Considerations in End-of-Life Care for Older Persons with Lifelong Disabilities
Douglas P. Olsen and Linda J. Keilman

Improving the Care of Women with Vulvovaginal Atrophy in Primary Care
Susan G. Wiers

Approaching Frailty in Primary Care
Deborah Dunn

Recognizing and Addressing Elder Abuse in the Primary Care Setting
Natalie R. Baker and Jennifer Kim

Women's Health

First-trimester Bleeding: Assessment, Diagnosis, and Management by the Primary Care Nurse Practitioner
Elizabeth Munoz and Heather Robbins

Women's Health Care for Incarcerated Women
Donna Jackson-Köhlin

Safe Medications in Primary Care of the Pregnant Woman: Update on the New Medication Classification System
Kathleen Danhausen and Taneesha Reynolds

Updates in Family Planning Care for Primary Care Practitioners
Neena Qasba and David Kattan

Pediatrics

The American Academy of Pediatrics Bright Futures Guidelines: An Update for Primary Care Clinicians
Imelda Reyes and Jeannie Rodriguez

Closing the Gap: Addressing Adversity and Promoting Early Childhood Development
Ashley Darcy Mahoney, Danielle G. Dooley, Nicole V. Davis, Michelle Stephens, and Olanrewaju O. Falusi

Transition of Health Care in Children with Chronic Health Conditions
Sharron Close, Susan Brasher, Amy Blumling, Amy Talboy, and Kristy Martyn

Immunization Schedule Updates for Children, Adolescents, and Adults
Kimberly R. Joo

ADVANCES IN FAMILY PRACTICE NURSING

ELSEVIER
MOSBY

PREFACE

Primary Care Nurse Practitioner Practice in a New Era

Check for updates

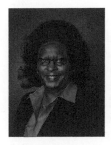
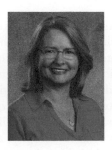
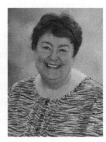
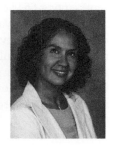

Geri C. Reeves, PhD, APRN, FNP-BC

Sharon L. Holley, DNP, CNM, FACNM

Linda J. Keilman, DNP, GNP-BC, FAANP

Imelda Reyes, DNP, MPH, APRN, CPNP-PC, FNP-BC, FAANP

Editors

P rimary care is a foundational element of the US health care system. Regular access to primary care is associated with receipt of more preventive services, early detection of health problems, and fewer preventable emergency department and hospital visits [1]. The Institute of Medicine's Committee on the Future of Primary Care defined primary care as: "The provision of integrated, accessible health services by clinicians who are accountable for addressing a large majority of personal health care needs, developing a sustained partnership with patients, and practicing in the context of family and community [2]$^{(p31)}$."

Converging trends characterized by an aging population, persistent health disparities, an expansion of access to primary care services under health care

https://doi.org/10.1016/j.yfpn.2019.02.001
2589-420X/19/© 2019 Published by Elsevier Inc.

reform, and the impending shortage of primary care physicians have chal-
lenged the ability of the US health care system to meet the growing demand
for primary care services [3]. Nurse practitioners (NPs) are a vital element of
the primary care workforce with a major role in making high-quality, patient-centered health care accessible to a broad range of consumers [4]. According to the 2018 American Academy of Nurse Practitioner National Nurse
Practitioner Sample Survey, 87.1% of NPs are certified in an area of primary
care, and 72.6% of all NPs deliver primary care. Family Nurse Practitioners
(FNPs), in particular, provide a significant portion of US primary care services,
representing 66.9% of all certified NPs [5].

The goal of Advances in Family Practice Nursing is to provide primary care
clinicians with relevant, evidence-based information on a wide range of topics,
in the areas of adult-gerontology, pediatric, and women's health. Each article
appearing in this issue of Family Practice Nursing supports this goal. Topics
include hypertension guidelines and medications, best practices in the management of major depression for older adults, travel health for older adults, ethical
considerations in end-of-life care for persons with lifelong disabilities,
improving the care of women with vulvovaginal atrophy, approaching frailty
in primary care, recognizing and addressing elder abuse in the primary care
setting, first-trimester bleeding, women's health care for incarcerated women,
safe medications in primary care of pregnant women, update on family planning, bright futures guideline update, promoting early brain and child development, transition from pediatric to adult care in chronic disease management,
and immunization schedule updates for children and adolescents.

Whether you're looking to update your knowledge in a particular area or to
read about the newest clinical advances to incorporate into your clinical practice, we trust this publication will provide useful and practical information that
will support the management of your patients.

Geri C. Reeves, PhD, APRN, FNP-BC
Vanderbilt University School of Nursing
461 21st Ave. South, 360 Frist Hall
Nashville, TN 37240, USA

E-mail address: geri.reeves@vanderbilt.edu

Sharon L. Holley, DNP, CNM, FACNM
Division of Midwifery & Community Health
Department of OB-Gyn at UMMS-Baystate
Baystate Medical Center
689 Chestnut Street
Springfield, MA 01199, USA

E-mail address: Sharon.holley@baystatehealth.org

Linda J. Keilman, DNP, GNP-BC, FAANP
Michigan State University
College of Nursing
1355 Bogue Street
A126 Life Science Building
East Lansing, MI 48824-1317, USA

E-mail address: keilman@msu.edu

Imelda Reyes, DNP, MPH, APRN, CPNP-PC, FNP-BC, FAANP
Emory University
Nell Hodgson Woodruff School of Nursing
1520 Clifton Road, Suite 432
Atlanta, GA 30322, USA

E-mail address: ireyes@emory.edu

References

[1] Phillips RL, Bazemore AW. Primary care and why it matters for US health system reform. Health Aff (Millwood) 2010;29(5):806–10.
[2] Donaldson MS, Yordy KD, Lohr KN, et al, editors. Institute of Medicine, Division of Health Care Services, Committee on the Future of Primary Care. Primary care: America's health in a new era. Washington, DC: National Academy Press; 1996. Available at: www.nap.edu/catalog.php?record_id=5152. Accessed January 29, 2019.
[3] Xue Y, Intrator O. Cultivating the role of nurse practitioners in providing primary care to vulnerable populations in an era of health-care reform. Policy, Politics, & Nursing Practice 2016;17(1):24–31.
[4] American Academy of Nurse Practitioners. Nurse Practitioners in Primary care. Available at: https://www.aanp.org/advocacy/advocacy-resource/position-statements/nurse-practitioners-in-primary-care. Accessed January 29, 2019.
[5] American Academy of Nurse Practitioners. NP fact sheet. Available at: https://www.aanp.org/about/all-about-nps/np-fact-sheet. Accessed January 29, 2019.

Adult/Geriatric

Advances in Family Practice Nursing 1 (2019) 1–13

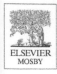

ADVANCES IN FAMILY PRACTICE NURSING

Individualized Approach to Hypertension Management Through Shared Decision Making

Katherine Dontje, PhD, FNP-BC*

College of Nursing, Michigan State University, East Lansing, MI 48824, USA

Keywords
- Hypertension • Shared decision-making • Primary care • Adults

Key points
- New guidelines for hypertension recommendations have changed diagnosis and treatment.
- Conflicting recommendations make determining a treatment plan difficult and support the use of shared decision making.
- A shared decision-making approach can facilitate patient-centered care.
- Decisions around hypertension treatment should be individualized and include focus on the patient's values and preferences.

INTRODUCTION

Hypertension (HTN) is one of the most common conditions seen in the primary care setting and in addition, is considered a modifiable risk factor for cardiovascular disease and stroke [1]. However, determining the diagnosis and treatment is challenging for primary care providers (PCP) because of inconsistent recommendations about target blood pressures [2]. PCPs need to review the evidence supporting the guidelines to individualize the recommendations for treatment. Making decisions about the most appropriate treatment for any individual patient is complex and requires understanding patient preferences and values as part of the decision-making process.

According to the National Quality Forum, using a shared decision-making (SDM) process is a standard of care for all patients [3]. SDM is the process

Disclosure: The author has no commercial or financial conflicts of interest and no funding sources.

*3155 Bogue St., Michigan State University, East Lansing, MI 48824. *E-mail address:* dontje@msu.edu

https://doi.org/10.1016/j.yfpn.2019.01.005

by which patients and the PCP work together to make treatment decisions. The use of an SDM model engages patients in treatment decisions and supports patient-centered care [4]. This process encourages the PCP to learn the individual patient's values, goals, and preferences while providing evidence-based recommendations. The combination of patient focus and evidence-based recommendations leads to the most appropriate treatment plan [4].

The Agency for Healthcare Research and Quality designed an approach to the SDM process (SHARE) that PCPs can apply to a variety of health conditions. The SHARE approach includes a 5-step process to engage patients in SDM: (1) *S*eek your patient's participation, (2) *H*elp your patient explore options, (3) *A*ssess your patient's values and preferences, (4) *R*each a decision, and (5) *E*valuate your patient's decision [5]. Unfortunately, according to research data, implementation of the SDM process has been uncommon in primary care [4]. Decisions around HTN treatment are complex and provide an ideal opportunity for providers to use this process.

PCPs identified the primary barrier to the SDM process as the extra time it takes to communicate with patients [4,6]. Yet, data show that it takes only a few more minutes to implement an SDM process within primary care [4]. PCPs are often pushed to see a large number of patients due to the fee-for-service reimbursement system that remains the main source of revenue. PCPs need to be aware of the potential benefits of the SDM process and consider how they can organize the office team members to create an efficient workflow. Another common concern about the SDM process is that patients may be reluctant to engage in the process of SDM. Research indicates that most patients want to participate in the decision-making process [4,6]. The use of an approach such as SHARE can help the PCP to engage the patient in the multiple decisions around management of HTN.

GUIDELINE

There are many decision points in diagnosing and treating patients with HTN. One of the most important decisions for the PCP is which guideline to follow. In the past year, the American College of Cardiology (ACC) and the American Heart Association (AHA) have published guidelines that differ significantly from previous recommendations for diagnosis and treatment of HTN. The 2017 ACC/AHA HTN guidelines classify all individuals regardless of age as having Stage 1 HTN if blood pressure levels are at or above 130/80 [7]. According to the 2017 ACC/AHA HTN recommendations, the normal blood pressure category includes individuals who have a blood pressure reading at or below 120/80, those between 120/80 and 129/80 are categorized as having an elevated blood pressure, 130 to 139/80 to 89 is Stage 1 HTN and greater than 140/90 is considered Stage 2 [8]. These guidelines do not address differences by age, so all individuals older than 18 have the same target blood pressures.

In contrast, previous guidelines had higher target levels for starting treatment, and age was a consideration in recommendations. The Seventh Report of the Joint National Committee on Prevention, Detection, Evaluation, and

Treatment of High Blood Pressure (JNC7) [9] classified individuals as having HTN if blood pressure levels were higher than 140/90 [10]. The JNC7 was followed by the 2014 Evidence-Based Guideline for the Management of High Blood Pressure in Adults, Eighth Joint National Committee (JNC8) guidelines [11]. The recommendations to indicate treatment for individuals younger than 60 at blood pressure readings higher than 140/90 and for older than 60 150/90 (Table 1) [9,11].

Additional recommendations for treatment of adults older than 60 have come from the 2017 guideline developed and published by the American College of Physicians (ACP) and the American Academy of Family Physicians (AAFP) [12]. The basis of these recommendations was a systematic review of the evidence focused on those older than 60. The ACP/AAFP guidelines recommend that individuals start medication when their systolic blood pressure reaches 150. These guidelines are important to consider, as they cover a significant percentage of those with HTN in primary care. According to the National Health and Nutrition Examination Survey data, approximately 76% of adults 65 to 74 and 82% of those 75 and older have HTN [8]. Using SDM with older adults involves assessing cardiac risk factors and comorbidities, providing information about recommendations, and discussing patient values before determining when to initiate HTN treatment.

GUIDELINE EVIDENCE

Evaluation of guidelines is important and understanding the level of evidence used to determine the guidelines is essential to making recommendations for HTN diagnosis and treatment. The 2017 ACC/AHA guidelines [7] are influenced heavily by the results of the Systolic Blood Pressure Intervention Trial (SPRINT) [13]. This trial conducted in the United States and Puerto Rico at 102 clinical sites had 2 arms: one in which the treatment goal was to achieve a systolic blood pressure of 135 to 139, and a second more intensive treatment

Table 1
Blood pressure categories from the seventh report of the Joint National Committee (JNC) to the 2017 American College of Cardiology (ACC) and the American Heart Association (AHA) Guidelines

SBP, mm Hg		DBP, mm Hg	JNC7	2017 ACC/AHA
<120	and	<80	Normal BP	Normal BP
120–129	and	<80	Prehypertension	High BP
130–139	or	80–89	Prehypertension	Stage 1 hypertension
140–159	or	90–99	Stage 1 hypertension	Stage 2 hypertension
≥160	or	≥100	Stage 2 hypertension	Stage 2 hypertension

Abbreviations: BP, blood pressure; DBP, diastolic BP; SBP, systolic BP.
Adapted from Cushman WC, Johnson KC. The 2017 U.S. hypertension guidelines: what is important for older adults? J Am Geriatr Soc 2018;66(6):1062–7.

group with a target goal of systolic blood pressure of 120 or lower. Participants were at least 50 years old, had an initial systolic blood pressure higher than 130, and were at increased risk for cardiovascular disease. It is important to note that exclusions included patients with diabetes and those with a prior stroke. The study ended early because of the significant differences noted between the 2 groups in outcome results. The main outcome of the trial was lower rates of both cardiovascular deaths and cardiovascular events in the group that maintained blood pressures at or below 120 systolic [13].

In contrast, the Action to Control Cardiovascular Risk in Diabetes (ACCORD) trial had identical systolic blood pressure targets of either less than 120 or 140 but did not find significant differences in cardiac outcomes [14]. The ACCORD trial was a multicenter randomized clinical trial. All patients in the trial were adults with a diagnosis of diabetes and were younger than 80. The design of the primary intervention was to evaluate if treating patients to achieve HgbA1c to normal levels (lower than 6) would decrease cardiovascular morbidity and mortality. The secondary aim of the trial was to evaluate if lower blood pressure and cholesterol levels would affect cardiac outcomes. Participants were randomized to receive intensive treatment for blood pressure (target of 120 systolic) or standard therapy for blood pressure (target systolic of 140 or less). The outcomes of this trial did not show a difference in the 2 blood pressure target arms in reduction of major cardiovascular events [15].

The ACP/AAFP guideline focused on recommendations for pharmacologic treatment of HTN in adults 60 years and older. The process used to develop these guidelines was a systematic review of randomized controlled trials. The purpose was to evaluate the benefits and harms of 2 different target blood pressures in this population on mortality and morbidity. The review focused on studies that evaluated patients with systolic blood pressure of 150 versus systolic pressure at or below 140 [12]. The evidence from the review led to 3 recommendations. First is to initiate pharmacologic treatment for patients older than 60 at a target blood pressure higher than 150 systolic and to treat to a target blood pressure below 150 systolic (supported by high-quality evidence). Second is that PCPs should intensify treatment for those patients with a history of stroke or transient ischemic attack to reach a target blood pressure goal of 140 systolic (supported by moderate-quality evidence). Third is to intensify pharmacologic treatment for those with high cardiovascular risk to a target goal of less than 140 (supported by low-quality evidence) [12]. This recommendation is for older adults and takes into consideration the risk/benefit of lower blood pressures in an adult population that also may be at increased risk for falls.

The PCP should be aware of some differences in the evidence used to determine recommendations that may have influenced the differences in target blood pressures. In review of the evidence from the SPRINT trial, it has been identified that measurement of blood pressures was through a very strict protocol by an automated measurement system. The use of this type of measurement may have resulted in blood pressure readings 10 to 15 points lower than blood pressure measurements in other studies [16]. Another consideration is the level of evidence related to patients' cardiac risk factors. The 2017 ACC/AHA recommendation to treat at a systolic blood pressure of 130 regardless of age is supported by high-level evidence for those individuals with cardiovascular disease or a greater than 10% 10-year atherosclerotic cardiovascular disease (ASCVD) risk, but for those with less than 10% arteriosclerotic vascular disease risk, the recommendation is based on observational data [8]. In addition, the ACC/AHA 2017 HTN guideline recommendation for treating to a diastolic blood pressure of 80 is based on expert opinion. Most high-level evidence on diastolic blood pressures recommends treatment to lower than 90 [8]. Yet, the choice made by the ACC/AHA guideline group was to recommend treating to a diastolic lower than 80. Reaching this target may require additional medication, which in patients with high risk for cardiac disease may outweigh the potential for side effects or potential medication interactions. In contrast, in someone with a lower cardiac risk who has a high potential for falls, the decision to add medications to achieve a blood pressures lower than 130/80 needs to be explored with the patient.

BLOOD PRESSURE MEASUREMENT

The accuracy of blood pressure readings used to diagnosis HTN is a consideration before diagnosis or treatment decisions [7,17] Several methods are available to measure blood pressure and each have pros and cons. The office blood pressure measurement (OBPM) uses either a manual or automated sphygmomanometer. To accurately obtain a blood pressure using this method, the ACC/AHA High Blood Pressure Guideline recommends a 6-step process that includes information on how the patient is prepared, proper technique, proper measurement, and documentation [7]. The process includes taking 2 or more blood pressures on 2 separate occasions before determining a diagnosis of HTN. The blood pressure is then determined using the average of these readings.

Patient self-monitoring of blood pressure has been shown to improve patient adherence and to lower blood pressure [18]. Self-monitoring also can help determine if a patient may have white coat or masked HTN. In white coat HTN, the blood pressure reading in the office is higher than blood pressures in their typical environment. In masked HTN, the blood pressure reading in the office is erroneously low. The accuracy of self-monitoring depends on patient knowledge of proper technique [19]. Patients are encouraged to record their blood pressures and to take the blood pressures at various times during the day. It is important to test the blood pressure equipment periodically for accuracy. The patient should bring in his or her cuff and compare it with the reading obtained in the office setting. The data from the self-monitoring of blood pressure can identify if there are significant variations from the OBPM and potentially prevent overtreatment.

The Canadian HTN Education Program Guidelines recommended the use of automated office blood pressure (AOBP) as the preferred method for determining blood pressure [20]. Research has shown AOBP in comparison with OBPM is a more accurate measurement of the patient's actual blood pressure [21]. The process involves leaving the patient in the examination room alone for 5 minutes and then the monitor takes 5 readings at prespecified intervals. This process decreases the incidence of white coat HTN but requires a specialized device that is not common in primary care offices.

The final option for measuring blood pressure is ambulatory blood pressure monitoring (ABPM). This method involves patients wearing a blood pressure cuff around their arm as they go about their regular activities for 24 hours. The digital monitor takes blood pressure measurements on scheduled intervals. The most accurate measurement of blood pressure is ABPM. Because of the high cost, ABPM is reserved for those patients who are not responding to medication or an individual suspected to have white coat HTN. The importance of accurate measurement of blood pressure should be discussed with the patient and a plan for which method to use should be agreed on before treatment decisions.

RISK FACTOR EVALUATION

Before starting treatment for HTN, the patient should have a thorough evaluation for modifiable risk factors. Smoking cessation is one of the key modifiable risk factors for HTN. Most primary care offices screen for smoking status but may not always take the time to develop a detailed plan for smoking cessation. The level of evidence to support this recommendation is high [7]. The challenge is to engage the patient in SDM about smoking cessation. Behavior change related to smoking requires the PCP to understand the patient's values and preferences and then assist the patient in making and maintaining change. Smoking cessation is often difficult for individuals and requires ongoing interaction with the PCP to find the best tools and resources for them to be successful.

Screening for recreational drugs and alcohol is highly recommended [7]. The use of a screening tool such as the Alcohol Use Disorders Identification Test (AUDIT) is one option to help identify individuals who drink more than the recommended levels of alcohol (1 drink for women and 2 for men) or those who may binge drink [22]. Validated screening tools also are available for recreational drug use. One concern about using these tools is the time it adds to the office visit. However, it is important not to base treatment recommendations on falsely high blood pressure. The PCP can use the SHARE process to seek the patient's participation, help the patient explore and understand the effects of alcohol and recreational drug use on blood pressure, and discuss options for assisting with decreasing alcohol or recreational drug use.

INTERVENTIONS

Recommendations for implementing healthy eating habits are something that can benefit all patients who have elevated blood pressure. The 2017 ACC/AHA guidelines recommend weight loss and a heart-healthy diet. The

Dietary Approaches to Stop Hypertension (DASH) eating plan was developed and tested in a multicenter randomized controlled study. Participants included individuals with diabetes and heart failure [23]. This eating plan emphasizes the following:

- Fruits and vegetables
- Whole grains
- Low-fat dairy products
- Increasing poultry, fish, legumes, and nuts
- Limiting red meat and sugar-sweetened beverages

The level of evidence to support a heart-healthy diet is high [24]. The 2017 ACC/AHA recommendations encourage dietary modifications before starting any medications for those in the categories of elevated blood pressure and Stage 1 HTN if the 10-year ASCVD risk is lower than 10% [7]. As part of the SDM process, the PCP should provide resources and support for patients to make behavioral change. Dietary modifications are difficult, and sharing information about reliable community-based resources for weight loss assistance with patients can assist the patient in making changes.

Dietary recommendations also address nutritional supplements. The 2017 ACC/AHA HTN guidelines recommend decreasing sodium intake to less than 1500 mg [7]. This level may be difficult for most individuals to accomplish. The Centers for Disease Control and Prevention recommendations are to reduce sodium intake to 2300 to 2400 mg daily intake [25]. Patients are often unfamiliar with hidden sources of sodium and may be consuming more sodium than they identify. It is important to discuss recommendations in relationship to individual dietary intake as it relates to culture and food choices. Potassium supplementation through dietary modifications is a recommended intervention [7]. The recommendation for daily potassium intake from the US Food and Drug Administration for an average adult is 4700 mg [26]. When discussing these recommendations, it can be helpful for the provider to provide a list of foods with sources of potassium (Table 2) and work with the patient to see how this level relates to their present intake.

Once a treatment plan is developed, helping the patient set reasonable goals is an essential component for making positive lifestyle change. One way to help the patient set specific goals is to use the SMART goals process (Specific, Measurable, Achievable, Reasonable, and Timely) [27]. This process engages the patient in determining small measurable and achievable goals. If the goal is to eat more fresh fruits and vegetables, the patient needs to explore barriers including knowledge level related to dietary recommendations and access to healthy foods [28]. Many individuals may not have transportation to grocery stores that provide an adequate supply of fresh fruits and vegetables at a reasonable price. It is important to address barriers to goal achievement and to provide information to patients to assist in making healthy food choices.

Patients with elevated blood pressures should be encouraged to engage in physical activity regularly. The benefits of regular physical activity include a

Table 2
Selected food sources of potassium

Food	Milligrams per serving	Percent of daily value
Apricots, dried, ½ cup	1101	31
Lentils, cooked, 1 cup	731	21
Prunes, dried, ½ cup	699	20
Squash, acorn, mashed, 1 cup	644	18
Raisins, ½ cup	618	18
Potato, baked, flesh only, 1 medium	610	17
Kidney beans, canned, 1 cup	607	17
Orange juice, 1 cup	496	14
Soybeans, mature seeds, boiled, ½ cup	443	13
Banana, 1 medium	422	12
Milk, 1%, 1 cup	366	10
Spinach, raw, 2 cups	334	10
Chicken breast, boneless, grilled, 3 ounces	332	9
Yogurt, fruit variety, nonfat, 6 ounces	330	9
Salmon, Atlantic, farmed, cooked, 3 ounces	326	9
Beef, top sirloin, grilled, 3 ounces	315	9
Tomato, raw, 1 medium	292	8
Soymilk, 1 cup	287	8
Broccoli, cooked, chopped, ½ cup	229	7
Cantaloupe, cubed, ½ cup	214	6
Turkey breast, roasted, 3 ounces	212	6
Asparagus, cooked, ½ cup	202	6
Apple, with skin, 1 medium	195	6
Cashew nuts, 1 ounce	187	5
Rice, brown, medium-grain, cooked, 1 cup	154	4
Tuna, light, canned in water, drained, 3 ounces	153	4
Coffee, brewed, 1 cup	116	3
Peanut butter, 1 tablespoon	90	3
Tea, black, brewed, 1 cup	88	3
Bread, whole-wheat, 1 slice	81	2
Egg, 1 large	69	2
Rice, white, medium-grain, cooked, 1 cup	54	2
Bread, white, 1 slice	37	1
Cheese, mozzarella, part skim, 1½ ounces	36	1

Adapted from National Institutes of Health: Office of dietary supplements potassium fact sheet for health professionals. 2018. Available at: https://ods.od.nih.gov/factsheets/Potassium-HealthProfessional/#h2. Accessed October 24, 2018.

decrease in atherosclerosis, increased cardiac function, decreased body fat, and decreased all-cause mortality from cardiovascular events [29]. Physical activity recommendations for lowering blood pressure are the same as for healthy adults. The PCP should assess the patient's level of exercise and encourage 30 to 40 minutes of aerobic physical activity approximately 3 to 4 times a week for a total of 90 to 150 minutes [7,29]. A systematic review done on effects of physical activity on lowering blood pressure found that even small amounts of physical activity on a consistent basis can make a difference in blood pressure [29]. It is important to talk with patients about a variety of ways to achieve increase in physical activity and the evidence behind the recommendation. As adults age, it is vital to continue to be active. As the PCP and the patient develop SMART goals for physical activity, it is helpful to understand available community resources and to offer information and alternatives to achieve these goals.

MEDICATION REVIEW

Recommendations are to obtain a complete medication history, which includes all prescribed medications, over-the-counter medications, and supplements used by the patient. Many medications elevate blood pressure. Those include but are not limited to the following:

- Antidepressants
- Systemic corticosteroids
- Nonsteroidal anti-inflammatory drugs
- Decongestants
- Herbal supplements (St. John's Wort)
- Recreational drugs (cocaine and methamphetamine) [7].

If medications are identified as a potential cause of the elevated blood pressure, a discussion should take place with the patient about the risks and benefits of stopping these medications and how this relates to treatment for HTN. Understanding the patient's preferences is important to making the shared decision about treatment. For example, the patient with depression may not be willing or able to change medications. The decision may be to add an antihypertensive medication to control the blood pressure within recommended levels.

RISK ASSESSMENT

Assessment of the patient for long-term cardiac risk has become a required step before determining the plan of care for HTN. The 2017 ACC/AHA HTN guidelines include consideration of a patient's risk factors before starting medications in Stage 1 HTN. The guidelines recommend the use of the 10-year ASCVD risk tool [7]. The ASCVD risk tool predicts the absolute 10-year risk for preventable ASCVD events (coronary death, nonfatal myocardial infarction, and fatal or nonfatal stroke) [30]. The risk tool uses information about the patient, including cholesterol levels, gender, age, systolic blood pressure, antihypertensive treatment use, diabetes mellitus history, and current smoking status. The developers of this tool used a pooled cohort equations model using data from several cohort studies funded by the National Heart, Lung, and Blood Institute to provide specific risk data for differences in gender and race [30]. However, validation of the tool was for patients between the ages of 40 and 79 years. The 10-year risk calculation is an important component of the information needed to discuss treatment recommendations with the patient.

In the 2017 ACC/AHA HTN guidelines, the recommendations for a patient diagnosed with Stage 1 HTN vary depending on the 10-year ASCVD risk score. If the risk is lower than 10%, recommendations are to advise lifestyle changes and monitoring. If a patient has a 10-year ASCVD risk of 10% or greater, the treatment recommendations are for medication and lifestyle interventions. Individuals diagnosed with HTN should have a urinalysis, basic metabolic panel, lipid profile, and 12-lead electrocardiogram before starting medication. If these are all normal, the decision of which medication to recommend requires a careful assessment of the patient's comorbidities and understanding the patient's values and preferences.

PHARMACOLOGIC TREATMENT

Both the ACA/AHA and the ACP/AAFP guidelines have similar recommendations for initial pharmacologic treatment. Previous guidelines had recommended several different medication classes as first-line treatment. The recent guidelines have removed beta-blockers as first-line therapy [7,12]. Recommendations for initial pharmacologic treatment for individuals in Stage I with an ASCVD risk of greater than 10% should be one of the following: thiazide diuretics, calcium channel blockers (CCBs), angiotensin-converting enzyme (ACE) inhibitors, or angiotensin II receptor blockers (ARBs). Recommendations discourage use of a combination of ACE inhibitors and ARBs together because of the potential harm, especially for patients who are at risk of vascular events or renal disease [7]. The decision of which medication to start first is impacted by potential side effects, such as increased urination, erectile dysfunction, and interactions with other medications. Patients should be aware of the potential side effects of each medication so as to choose the most appropriate medication. If the patient does not have a clear understanding of side effects, there is a risk the patient may stop the medication on his or her own without considering other options. Discussing with patients the importance of calling the office before stopping medications can prevent some miscommunication and lack of treatment due to stoppage of medications.

The next step in the SDM process is to use the evaluation component of the SHARE model [5]. Evaluation requires discussing with the patient the importance of follow-up and sharing with the patient the target blood pressure level. The ACC/AHA guideline recommends that patients follow-up monthly until blood pressure levels meet the target goal [7]. Each of these visits should include evaluation of all the treatment decisions made with the patient. The review includes the SMART goals for medication, dietary modifications, physical activity, smoking cessation, or changes in recreational drug use. Once the patient achieves the target goals, he or she should follow-up every 3 to 6 months for monitoring and maintenance support of lifestyle changes.

In patients with comorbidities, the recommendations for medication therapy vary depending on the comorbidity [7]. For example, if the patient has diabetes or chronic kidney disease, the recommendation is to use an ACE inhibitor or ARB as first line. If the patient is African American, the recommendation is to start a thiazide diuretic followed by CCB. ACE inhibitors and beta-blockers are not as effective in the African American population [31]. If the patient's blood pressure fails to respond to more than 3 medications at optimal doses, including a diuretic, they are considered treatment resistant and require further evaluation [7]. One of the first steps before assuming blood pressure is treatment resistant is to have a conversation with the patient and confirm the patient's ability to follow recommendations for lifestyle modification and explore medication adherence. Recommendations for additional treatment of resistant HTN and other comorbid conditions are available in the 2017 ACC/AHA guidelines document and are beyond the scope of this discussion.

DISCUSSION

Blood pressure treatment options are determined based on the best evidence available at this time. The future will include the use of precision medicine or personalized medicine that can provide a tailored approach to therapeutic interventions. Precision medicine requires the identification of specific genetic factors as well as environmental influences that precede the diagnosis of HTN. Currently, researchers have not been able to identify these related to HTN. Chronic conditions that have a complex network of genetic and environmental factors that influence the development of the condition need more research [32]. The focus of new therapies will be on early prevention measures and the potential to develop targeted drug therapy. Researchers are making progress toward this goal; however, due to the large number of genetic variants, it has not been possible to develop targeted therapies [32]. As a result, at this time, PCPs rely on guidelines developed based on the best evidence available. The complexity of these recommendations and the conflicting recommendations for diagnosis and treatment make it essential to work with the patient to make treatment decisions using an SDM model. Engaging patients in treatment decisions increases the chance that patients will follow through with the mutually agreed on plan. Patients who have their HTN treated to the target blood pressure goals have a decreased risk of morbidity and mortality related to cardiovascular conditions. The key factor is to discuss the options with the patient and through SDM determine the best individualized plan available for each patient.

References

[1] Benjamin EJ, Virani SS, Callaway CW, et al. Heart disease and stroke statistics—2018 update: a report from the American Heart Association. Circulation 2018;137(12):e67–492.

[2] Wang S, Khera R, Das SR, et al. Usefulness of a simple algorithm to identify hypertensive patients who benefit from intensive blood pressure lowering. Am J Cardiol 2018;122(2): 248–54.

[3] National Quality Forum. National Quality Forum Action Brief. Shared Decision making: A standard of care for all patients. October 2017. Available at: https://www.qualityforum.org/Publications/2017/10/NQP_Shared_Decision_Making_Action_Brief.aspx. Accessed February 8, 2019.

[4] Stiggelbout AM, Pieterse A, De Haes J. Shared decision making: concepts, evidence, and practice. Patient Educ Couns 2015;98(10):1172–9.

[5] Agency for Healthcare Research and Quality. The share approach 2014. Available at: https://www.ahrq.gov/professionals/education/curriculum-tools/shareddecisionmaking/index.html. Accessed August 29, 2018.

[6] Légaré F, Thompson-Leduc P. Twelve myths about shared decision making. Patient Educ Couns 2014;96(3):281-6.

[7] Whelton PK, Carey RM. The 2017 American College of Cardiology/American Heart Association clinical practice guideline for high blood pressure in adults. JAMA Cardiol 2018;3(4):352-3.

[8] Cushman WC, Johnson KC. The 2017 US hypertension guidelines: what is important for older adults? J Am Geriatr Soc 2018;66(6):1062-7.

[9] Chobanian AV, Bakris GL, Black HR, et al. The seventh report of the Joint National Committee on prevention, detection, evaluation, and treatment of high blood pressure. JAMA 2003;289(19):2560-72.

[10] Armstrong C. JNC8 guidelines for the management of hypertension in adults. Am Fam Physician 2014;90(7):503-4.

[11] James PA, Oparil S, Carter BL, et al. 2014 evidence-based guideline for the management of high blood pressure in adults: report from the panel members appointed to the eighth Joint National Committee (JNC 8). JAMA 2014;311(5):507-20.

[12] Qaseem A, Wilt TJ, Rich R, et al. Pharmacologic treatment of hypertension in adults aged 60 years or older to higher versus lower blood pressure targets: a clinical practice guideline from the American College of Physicians and the American Academy of Family Physicians. Ann Intern Med 2017;166(6):430-7.

[13] Muntner P, Carey RM, Gidding S, et al. Potential US population impact of the 2017 ACC/AHA high blood pressure guideline. Circulation 2018;137(2):109-18.

[14] Wright JT Jr, Williamson JD, Whelton PK, et al. A randomized trial of intensive versus standard blood-pressure control. N Engl J Med 2015;373(22):2103-16.

[15] Gerstein HC, Miller ME, Byington RP, et al. Effects of intensive glucose lowering in type 2 diabetes. N Engl J Med 2008;358(24):2545-59.

[16] van der Leeuw J, Visseren FL, Woodward M, et al. Predicting the effects of blood pressure-lowering treatment on major cardiovascular events for individual patients with type 2 diabetes mellitus: results from action in diabetes and vascular disease: preterax and diamicron MR controlled evaluation. Hypertension 2015;65(1):115-21.

[17] Brunstrom M, Carlberg B. Association of blood pressure lowering with mortality and cardiovascular disease across blood pressure levels: a systematic review and meta-analysis. JAMA Intern Med 2018;178(1):28-36.

[18] Siu AL. Screening for high blood pressure in adults: US preventive services task force recommendation statement. Ann Intern Med 2015;163(10):778-86.

[19] Stergiou GS, Kario K, Kollias A, et al. Home blood pressure monitoring in the 21st century. J Clin Hypertens (Greenwich) 2018;20(7):1116-21.

[20] McManus RJ, Mant J, Haque MS, et al. Effect of self-monitoring and medication self-titration on systolic blood pressure in hypertensive patients at high risk of cardiovascular disease: the TASMIN-SR randomized clinical trial. JAMA 2014;312(8):799-808.

[21] Leung AA, Nerenberg K, Daskalopoulou SS, et al. Hypertension Canada's 2016 Canadian hypertension education program guidelines for blood pressure measurement, diagnosis, assessment of risk, prevention, and treatment of hypertension. Can J Cardiol 2016;32(5):569-88.

[22] Kaner EF, Beyer FR, Muirhead C, et al. Effectiveness of brief alcohol interventions in primary care populations. Cochrane Database Syst Rev 2018;(2):CD004148.

[23] Tyson CC, Nwankwo C, Lin P-H, et al. The dietary approaches to stop hypertension (DASH) eating pattern in special populations. Curr Hypertens Rep 2012;14(5):388-96.

[24] Saneei P, Salehi-Abragoel A, Esmalill A, et al. Influence of Dietary Approaches to Stop Hypertension (DASH) diet on blood pressure: a systematic review and meta-analysis on randomized controlled trials. Nutr Metab Cardiovasc Dis 2014;24(12):1253-61.

[25] Suckling RJ, He FJ, Markandu ND, et al. Modest salt reduction lowers blood pressure and albumin excretion in impaired glucose tolerance and type 2 diabetes mellitus: a randomized double-blind trial. Hypertension 2016;67(6):1189–95.

[26] Tichelaar J, Uil den SH, Antonini NF, et al. A 'SMART' way to determine treatment goals in pharmacotherapy education. Br J Clin Pharmacol 2016;82(1):280–4.

[27] Rifai L, Silver MA. A review of the DASH diet as an optimal dietary plan for symptomatic heart failure. Prog Cardiovasc Dis 2016;58(5):548–54.

[28] Sharman JE, La Gerche A, Coombes JS. Exercise and cardiovascular risk in patients with hypertension. Am J Hypertens 2015;28(2):147–58.

[29] Goff DC Jr, Lloyd-Jones DM, Bennett G, et al. 2013 ACC/AHA guideline on the assessment of cardiovascular risk: a report of the American College of Cardiology/American Heart Association Task Force on Practice Guidelines. J Am Coll Cardiol 2014;63(25 Pt B):2935–59.

[30] Carnethon MR, Pu J, Howard G, et al. Cardiovascular health in African Americans: a scientific statement from the American Heart Association. Circulation 2017;136(21):e393–423.

[31] Patel RS, Masi S, Taddei S. Understanding the role of genetics in hypertension. Eur Heart J 2017;38(29):2309–12.

[32] Manunta P, Ferrandi M, Cusi D, et al. Personalized therapy of hypertension: the past and the future. Curr Hypertens Rep 2016;18(3):24.

Advances in Family Practice Nursing 1 (2019) 15–32

ADVANCES IN FAMILY PRACTICE NURSING

ELSEVIER
MOSBY

Best Practices in the Management of Major Depression for Older Adults in Primary Care

George Byron Peraza-Smith, DNP, APRN, GNP-BC, GS-C, CNE, FAANP*, Teresa Kiresuk, DNP, APRN, AGPCNP-C¹

College of Nursing and Public Health, South University, Savannah, GA, USA

Keywords

- Depression • Older adult • Vulnerable • Patient health questionnaire-2 (PHQ-2)
- Patient health questionnaire-9 (PHQ-9)

Key points

- Depression in late life is often underrecognized and undertreated in older adults in part because of older adults' and primary care providers' misconceptions about aging.
- Patient Health Questionnaire-2, Patient Health Questionnaire-9, and Geriatric Depression Scale are commonly used depression screens in primary care.
- As with younger cohorts, there are effective treatments for depression in older adults.

INTRODUCTION

Depression is often underrecognized and undertreated in older adults. Many primary care providers (PCPs), caregivers, and older adults themselves falsely believe that depression is just a fact of getting older; that depression is something older adults have to live with in later life; and that depression is an expected burden that comes with age and loss. However, depression is not an

Disclosure Statement: The authors have no disclosure of any relationship with a commercial company that has a direct financial interest in the subject matter or materials discussed in this article or with a company making a competing product.

¹Present address: 984 Paker Avenue, Roseville, MN 55113.

*Corresponding author. South University, 4401 North Himes Avenue, Tampa, FL 33614-7095. E-mail address: gperaza-smith@southuniversity.edu

https://doi.org/10.1016/j.yfpn.2018.11.001

age-related change and is not an expected part of getting older. Assessment and management of depression in older adults are essential skills for nurse practitioners (NP) in primary care. However, PCPs may encounter significant challenges in identifying and managing depression in older adults. The identification of depression may be hindered because of symptoms of depression masking as vague complaints or somatic symptoms. Depression in older adults is often exacerbated by multimorbid chronic conditions and may be compounded from continuous losses in all spheres of an older person's life: function, health, dependence, and friends/family/peers. Understanding the potential burden of depression in late life is an important step toward recognition and effective treatment of depression for older adults.

Epidemiology

Between 2017 and 2036, there will be an estimated 10,000 individuals in the United States turning 65 years old every day; that equals an individual turning 65 years old every 8 seconds [1]. The proportion of the US population that is 65 years or older will drastically change from 39.7 million (13%) in 2010 to more than 67 million (18%) by 2030 [2]. It is projected that the population of people aged 65 and older will climb to 98.2 million in 2060. One in 4 individuals in the United States will be 65 years old, whereas 19.7 million older adults will be aged 85 or older [3]. In the United States, life expectancy at birth increased from 72.6 years in 1975 to 78.8 years in 2015. For men, life expectancy increased from 68.8 years in 1975 to 76.3 years in 2015, and for women, life expectancy increased from 76.6 years in 1975 to 81.2 years in 2015 [4].

The aging population will place increasing expectations and demands on the health care system. In 2016, the health expenditures in the United States grew 4.3% to 3.3 trillion or $10,348 per person and accounted for 17.9% of the gross domestic product. Medicare spending grew 3.6% to $672.1 billion or 20% of the total national health expenditures [5]. Medicare spending was 15% of total federal spending in 2017 and is projected to increase to 18% by 2028 [6]. Older adults made up 13% of the US population in 2010 but accounted for 34% of the health care cost [5]. The Centers for Medicare and Medicaid Services estimates there will be 81 million beneficiaries in 2030 [7].

By 2030, it is projected that more than 15 million older adults, or one in 5 older adults over the age of 60 years, will be diagnosed with a mental disorder [8]. In the United States, an estimated 16.2 million adults or 6.7% have had one major depressive episode in their lifetime [9]. The prevalence of a major depressive episode was 4.8% among adults 50 years and older [9]. Between 5.6 and 8 million, or nearly one in 5 older adults in the United States, have one or more mental health and/or substance abuse conditions [10]. It is estimated that more than 13% of older adults have experienced depression [11]. Depression is more common in older women than older men, but older men seek treatment for depression at a lower rate [12]. Older adults with late life depression are at higher risk for developing dementia and have increased morbidity and mortality from cardiovascular diseases, such as hypertension, coronary heart disease, and diabetes [13]. Depression costs billions of dollars each year from increased emergency and office visits, increased drug use, higher risk for alcohol and substance use, and increased length of hospitalizations [13]. The US population is getting older with multiple comorbid chronic conditions that include mental health and substance abuse issues. Improving the PCP's awareness of the depression rates among older adults, and the fact that there are effective treatments for depression, may lead to earlier interventions and improved outcomes for older adults with depression.

CLINICAL FEATURES AND ASSESSMENT

Depression is not a normal aging change or an expected part of aging. Depression is a medical condition that can usually be treated effectively. Depression in older adults is often unrecognized or misdiagnosed leading to delayed treatment and unnecessary suffering. Older adults many times have multiple medical conditions that take precedence over their mental health needs. PCPs often misunderstand the negative impact of untreated mental conditions on the overall outcome and health of the older adult. Some PCPs mistakenly believe that if they take care of the physical disorders, the mental disorders will resolve on their own. The older adult should be viewed and treated from a holistic perspective with the understanding that the mind and body work in concert for achieving and maintaining overall health.

Depression affects every domain of the older adult's life. Untreated depression may lead to loss of independent function, social isolation, cognitive impairment, emotional distress, delirium, and poor health outcomes. Untreated depression can lead to a shortened life expectancy and cause untold mental and physical anguish. Delayed detection and treatment of depression may impede the older adult from reaching remission and lead to treatment resistance [14,15]. Depression can lead to significant family conflicts and disruption. The conflicts can stem from unrealistic expectations or misinterpretation of symptoms by the family and/or significant others in the older adult's life. The older adult may become withdrawn, disengaged, disinterested, isolative, agitated, or anxious. This change often creates disharmony between older adults with depression and others, leading to further isolation and discourse.

The *Diagnostic and Statistical Manual of Mental Disorders* (fifth edition) (*DSM-5*) [16] defines depression as consisting of 5 or more of the following symptoms that must have been present in the same 2-week period that is a change from usual functioning. At least one symptom must be either a depressed mood or loss of interest:

1. Depressed or sad mood for most of the time of the day as indicated by self-report (eg, describe feeling depressed, sad, or blue) through observations made by others (eg, tearful, sad facial expression, closed posture).
2. Marked diminished interest or anhedonia in all, or almost all, activities most of the day and nearly every day (eg, indicated by self-report or through observation by others).

3. Significant weight loss when not dieting or weight gain (eg, a change of more than 5% of body weight in a month or from previous office visit), or decrease or increase in appetite nearly every day.
4. Insomnia or hypersomnia nearly every day.
5. Psychomotor agitation or retardation nearly every day (observable by others, not merely subjective feelings of restlessness or being slowed down).
6. Fatigue or loss of energy nearly every day.
7. Feelings of worthlessness or excessive or inappropriate guilt (which may be delusional) nearly every day (not merely self-reproach or guilt about being sick).
8. Diminished ability to think or concentrate, or indecisiveness, nearly every day (either by subjective account or as observed by others).

Recurrent thoughts of death (not just fear of dying), recurrent suicidal ideation without a specific plan, or a suicide attempt or a specific plan for committing suicide (see Diagnostic Criteria for Major Depressive Disorder and Depressive Episodes, https://www.psnpaloalto.com/wp/wp-content/uploads/2010/12/Depression-Diagnostic-Criteria-and-Severity-Rating.pdf).

In order to meet the definition of depression, symptoms must have caused significant distress or impairment in social, occupational, or other important areas of functioning. The depression symptoms cannot be attributed to the physiologic effects of a substance or to another psychiatric or medical condition. In older adults, other conditions or potential causes for depression symptoms can masquerade as depression and must be ruled out before diagnosing depression (Box 1). Once a complete history and physical examination have been completed, certain diagnostic studies may be indicated to rule out potential medical causes for depression symptoms (Box 2). The organization of the

Box 1: Rule out conditions for depression in older adults

- Dementia
- Chronic, persistent pain
- Anxiety
- Sleep disturbances
- Anemia
- Diabetes
- Hypothyroidism
- Stroke
- Substance use or abuse
- Delirium
  - Dehydration
  - Infection
  - Metabolic imbalance
  - Medication side effect or adverse event

Box 2: Possible diagnostic testing for depression
- Complete blood count
- Comprehensive metabolic panel
- Thyroid function studies
- Vitamin B12 levels
- C-reactive protein
- Vitamin D-25(OH) D level
- Blood and urine toxicology
- Electrocardiogram

International Classification of Diseases, Tenth Revision, Clinical Modifications codes for major depressive disorders are based on severity of the depression, the presence of any associated symptoms, and whether the episode or episodes of depression are in partial or full remission (see F32 Major depressive disorder, single episode, http://www.mentalhealthamerica.net/preventing-suicide-older-adults and F33 Major depressive disorder, recurrent, http://www.mentalhealth-america.net/preventing-suicide-older-adults).

Assessment

Depression in older adults, also called late life depression, is depression that occurs after the age of 60 years. The onset of depression in older adults can start at any time before or after turning 60 years of age. Nearly two-thirds of older adults with depression will present to a PCP [17]. The stigma of having a mental disorder or condition prevents many older adults from seeking treatment or sharing symptoms with providers. Most older adults prefer to see their familiar PCP rather than seek out a mental health specialist. In a primary care setting, there may be unique challenges to assessing and diagnosing depression in older adults. Older adults tend to focus on somatic symptoms or bodily complaints rather than the psychological distress of depression. Many older adults see depression as a weakness of character. Older adults are either consciously or subconsciously more accepting of bodily complaints that are equated to a physical cause of distress over a diagnosis of a depression disorder that is equated to a mental failing.

When assessing for depression in older adults, the PCP should first convey a sense of caring and presence. Assessing depression in older adults takes patience and cannot be completed effectively within a 12-minute office visit. In primary care, the older adults need to feel that they can trust the provider. Fostering the PCP/patient relationship is critical to both effectively assessing and treating the older adult. Older adults many times do not have the words to effectively communicate the symptoms of depression. The PCP often has to distinguish between the medical comorbid symptoms or the medication adverse effects from the symptoms caused by depression. When at all possible, obtaining the perspective of the family and other significant individuals may help the older adult better realize the impact of the symptoms on their daily lives.

Assessment tools

There are many instruments used in practice to screen and assess for depression. The 3 commonly used instruments in primary care with older adults are the Patient Health Questionnaire-2 (PHQ-2), the Patient Health Questionnaire-9 (PHQ-9), and the Geriatric Depression Scale (GDS). The PHQ-2 is generally used as a screen and includes the first 2 questions from the PHQ-9 that inquires about the frequency of depressed mood and anhedonia over the past 2 weeks [18]. According to the *DSM-5*, the symptom of depressed mood or loss of interest must have been present for 2 weeks with an additional 4 symptoms present to be diagnosed with depression [16]. Answering "yes" to either depressed mood or anhedonia on the PHQ-2 would lead to further screening with the PHQ-9 or the GDS in older adults.

The PHQ-9 is a screen of depression symptoms over the last 2-week period. The instrument has 9 items and uses a Likert-type scale from 0 (not at all) to 3 (nearly every day) with higher scores indicating higher levels of depressive symptoms. The Cronbach alpha for the PHQ-9 is 0.86 [18]. Scores range from 0 to 27, and levels of depression severity fall into 4 depression levels: 0 to 4 (minimal), 5 to 9 (mild), 10 to 14 (moderate), and 15 or greater (moderately severe or severe) depression. The cutoff score for depression with the PHQ-9 is a total score of 10. The instrument is easy to administer as a self-report or interview format.

The GDS screens for depression in older adults from over the last week. The instrument has 15 items and uses a dichotomous scale with "Yes" denoting that the indicator was present and "No" denoting the indicator was not present with higher scores suggesting higher severity of depression. The Cronbach alpha for the GDS is 0.84 [19]. Scores range from 0 to 15. Scores of 0 to 4 are considered normal (depending on age, education, and complaints); 5 to 8 indicate mild depression; 9 to 11 indicate moderate depression; and 12 to 15 indicate severe depression. The instrument is easy to administer as a self-report or interview format.

Suicide risk

Suicide rates across the United States are on the increase, whereby suicide is the 10th leading cause of death. In 2016, the highest suicide rate (19.72/100,000) was among adults between 45 and 54 years of age. The second highest rate (18.98/100,000) occurred in those 85 years or older [3]. Older white men have the highest suicide rate at 48.7 per 100,000 suicides in the United States [8]. Risk factors and warning signs for suicide in older adults include depression and other mental health problems, substance use problems, physical illness, disability, chronic pain, or social isolation (see Preventing suicide in older adults, http://www.mentalhealthamerica.net/preventing-suicide-older-adults).

When assessing for suicidal risk, it is important for PCPs to listen and explore the feelings and thinking of the older adult. Asking the older adult if he or she is having thoughts of ending their life or of suicide conveys attentiveness and caring. Asking about thoughts of suicide will not cause the older adult to think or want to commit suicide nor will the older adult be offended. Asking the direct questions on suicide will communicate to the older adult that you see the emotional pain. Asking about suicide communicates that the PCP understands and wants to help. Potential questions to ask in assessing the older adults thinking on suicide include the following:

- Have you been having thoughts that your life is not worth living?
- Have you been having thoughts of killing yourself?
- Have you felt that you or your family would be better off without you?
- Do you wish you were dead?
- If you didn't wake up this morning, would that be ok with you?

Just because someone may have thoughts of harming or killing themselves does not necessarily mean they are actually going to end their life. However, older adults are more likely to attempt suicide if they have a specific plan and have available lethal means for carrying out the suicide. It is important to ask the questions on suicide risk. The PCP may be the only health care professional for an older adult. Asking the questions could save a life.

VULNERABLE GROUPS
Orphan or loneliness
An increasing number of adults are entering older age alone and disconnected from their families and community. An "elder orphan" is a term coined for older adults who are socially and/or physically isolated, without any available known family member, designated surrogate, or caregiver for support [20]. An estimated 22% of older adults 65 years and older is at risk of becoming orphan [21]. These older adults become orphan for reasons related to their own dysfunctional life choices or due to unforeseen circumstances. The older adult orphan may have become ostracized from family and friends. Many have multiple chronic conditions and functional limitations that lead to further isolation.

Older adult orphans are at risk for loneliness and depression. Loneliness is the discrepancy between desired and real social relations and engagement [22]. Research has indicated that loneliness may be more hazardous to depression than social isolation alone [23]. Cacioppo and Cacioppo [24] found a strong association between loneliness and depression among older adults. It is intuitive that depression and loneliness would occur together; however, many PCPs fail to consider loneliness' impact on the treatment of depression.

Substance abuse
Substance abuse in the United States has become a national crisis. In primary care, substance and/or alcohol abuse are often unrecognized and undertreated in older adults. There are an estimated 2.5 million older adults in the United

States who have a substance use disorder [25]. The number of older adults older than 50 years old with a substance abuse problem is predicted to double from 2.5 million in 1999 to 5 million in 2020 [26]. Many PCPs are not aware of the risk for alcohol and substance abuse among older populations. The CAGE Questions Adapted to Include Drug Use (CAGE-AID) screen provides a quick assessment of the potential for alcohol and substance abuse and can be used in primary care. The CAGE-AID screen is derived from the 4 questions of the tool: cut down (Have you ever felt you ought to cut down on your drinking or drug use?); annoyed (Have people annoyed you by criticizing your drinking or drug use?); guilty (Have you felt bad or guilty about your drinking or drug use?), and eye-opener (Have you ever had a drink or used drugs first thing in the morning to steady your nerves or to get rid of a hangover [eye-opener]?) [27]. The cutoff for the CAGE-AID is 2 positive responses; however, it is recommended for PCPs to lower the threshold to one positive response to reduce the chance of missing potential alcohol and drug abusers [28].

Poverty

An increasing number of older adults are finding themselves in poverty; they are struggling to pay for a place to live and for money to buy food. The Social Security and Medicaid safety net programs continue to shrink, causing some older adults to make tough life choices, such as choosing between eating and paying for medications or choosing to have a roof over their head and seeking medical treatment. Nearly 1 in 5 older adults approaching retirement have no retirement savings at all with 7.1 million adults aged 65 and older living in poverty [29]. Poverty negatively impacts the older adults' ability to seek effective treatment of depression. Effective depression treatment requires the older adult to continuously take medication and participate in some form of therapy. Even when depression is identified in older adults experiencing poverty, they are unable to access or maintain effective treatments for depression. The PCP must be aware of the unique challenges faced by older adults in poverty. The PCP can assist the older adult to access community specific services for older adults in poverty.

Lesbian, gay, bisexual, transgender, queer/questioning

The definitions of lesbian, gay, bisexual, transgender, queer/questioning (LGBT) vary widely and can be defined as the population of sexual and gender minorities, whereas the LGBTQ+ acronym attempts to be a more inclusive term for sexual and gender minorities. There are an estimated 2.4 to 4 million lesbian, gay, bisexual, and transgender (LGBT) adults over the age 50 years in the United States with a projection of more than 5 million LGBT older adults by 2030 [30]. This number does not include those who are questioning their sexuality or those who consider themselves sexually fluid. However, the older adult population is more likely to hold the traditional views of sexual identity and tend to identify as LGBT. The incidences of depression, anxiety, and suicidal risk are 2 to 3 times higher than the general population [31].

LGBTQ+ older adults often experience trepidation when seeking health care services due to a fear of being rejected and negatively judged by the PCP [32].

COMORBID CONDITIONS

Many physical medical conditions have a high prevalence of concomitant depression. Conversely, untreated depression can present with multiple physical and somatic symptoms that can be mistaken for physical illness. Depression occurring with a combined physical illness has higher mortality rates than either depression or physical illness alone [33]. Patients who have a physical diagnosis whereby there is significant limitation to functional status, high levels of pain, chronicity, rapid progression of the disease, and/or multiple physical diagnoses have higher incidence of concomitant depression. The risk for depression development is highest in the first 2 years following diagnosis of chronic physical medical illness [33].

It can be challenging to differentiate depression from other physical illness. Symptoms commonly seen in depression (fatigue, lack of energy, poor concentration, weight loss, pain) can often be the first sign of a physical illness, such as cerebrovascular conditions, cardiovascular conditions, diabetes, malignancies, and thyroid disorders. Depression is also associated with many of the medications used to treat illnesses that occur more frequently in older adults [34]. Common medical-related medications include beta-blockers, corticosteroids, calcium channel blockers, varenicline (Chantix), benzodiazepines, and medications with high anticholinergic properties can cause depression, or symptoms of depression (Table 1). Physical illness can contribute to feelings of helplessness, decreased or loss of self-worth and identity, inability to participate in activities of work or leisure, as well as a sense of hopelessness regarding quality of life and hopes of the future [35]. Table 2 identifies common diagnoses that are highly associated with depression.

Depression, when present at the onset of physical illness, is associated with higher medical mortality from myocardial infarction, stroke, and nursing home admission. Conversely, successful treatment of depression is associated with improved medical mortality [36]. Depression has been associated with higher health care utilization, lower rates of treatment compliance, and higher rates of poor health habits, such as poor diet and lack of exercise. These behaviors contribute to higher health care costs with poorer outcomes for treatment of medical conditions highly associated with depression. A cascade of events can follow with poor functional status occurring with or leading to depression. These events in turn may lead to further social isolation, disability, and functional status decline. Health care payers, including federally funded programs like Medicare and Medicaid, have introduced financial incentives for providers and facilities to identify and manage depression in older adults.

When illness does not respond to treatment as expected, or if some symptoms improve but others like fatigue and chronic pain do not, the PCP should suspect depression. Patients who are reluctant to participate in treatment of their physical illness, or do not engage with their PCP, may also have

Table 1
Drug classifications that may contribute to depression in older adults

Drug classification	Agents
Cardiovascular	• ACE inhibitors
	• Calcium channel blockers
	• Digitoxin
	• Hydralazine
	• Methyldopa
	• Propranolol
	• Reserpine
	• Thiazide diuretics
	• Zolamide diuretics
	• Clonidine
Antiparkinson	• Amantadine
	• Bromocriptine
	• Levodopa
Stimulants	• Caffeine
	• Methylphenidate
	• Amphetamines (when withdrawing)
Anti-infectives	• Ampicillin
	• Cyclosporine
	• Dapsone
	• Ganciclovir
	• Griseofulvin
	• Isoniazid
	• Interferon
	• Metronidazole
	• Nitrofurantoin
	• Penicillin G
	• Streptomycin
	• Sulfonamides
	• Tetracycline
	• Trimethoprim
Hormones	• Glucocorticoids
	• Anabolic steroids
Antipsychotics	• Haloperidol
Anxiolytics	• Benzodiazepines
Sedative and hypnotics	• Barbiturates
	• Chloral hydrate
Anticonvulsants	• Phenobarbital
	• Phenytoin
	• Primidone
	• Vigabatrin
Anti-inflammatory	• Nonsteroidal anti-inflammatory drugs

underlying depression. It is important that PCPs consider manifestations of physical symptoms as being related to underlying physical illness, depression, or both.

Depression can be particularly difficult to diagnose in the presence of dementia. The symptoms of dementia (such as social withdrawal, loss of interest in activities, flat or depressed affect, appetite changes, emotional

Table 2
Physical diagnoses that are highly associated with depression

Neurologic disorders	• Dementias
	  ○ Vascular
	  ○ Ischemic
	  ○ Degenerative
	• Seizure disorders
	• Intracranial lesions
	• Parkinson disease
	• Stroke
	  ○ Ischemic
	  ○ Vascular

Malignancies	• Pancreas • Lung
Endocrine	• Diabetes mellitus • Thyroid disorders • Hyperparathyroidism
Cardiac disorders	• Coronary heart disease • Myocardial infarction
Autoimmune disorders	• Multiple sclerosis • Rheumatoid arthritis • Scleroderma • Lupus • Muscular dystrophies
Vitamin & mineral deficiencies	• B12 • Folic acid • Thiamin • Vitamin D • Iron

fluctuations, sleep disruption) can be present in both dementia and depression. It is easy for the PCP to miss or delay the diagnosis of depression for patients who have dementia, especially if there is already significant cognitive loss. Conversely, it may be easy to miss or delay the diagnosis of dementia in the presence of depression when the cognitive changes are not advanced or clearly present. The National Institute of Mental Health (NIMH) has identified diagnostic criteria for depression in patients with dementia. The NIMH published provisional diagnostic criteria for depression in Alzheimer disease is identified (Box 3).

MANAGEMENT

Treatment of depression in older adults can be challenging. A multifaceted, multidisciplinary approach that is targeted to individual patient disease presentation is the most successful and challenging. Factors to consider include treatment setting, severity of the depression, prior history of depression, underlying medical diagnoses, underlying pharmacotherapy issues, risk for suicide, patient acceptance of the diagnosis, family support, and patient acceptance of both pharmacologic and nonpharmacologic measures. Indications for inpatient

Box 3: National Institute of Mental Health provisional diagnostic criteria for depression in Alzheimer disease

1. Three (or more) of the following symptoms must be present during the same 2-week period and represent a change from previous functioning. At least one of the symptoms must either be 1) depressed mood or 2) decreased positive affect or pleasure

    a. Clinically significant depressed mood

    b. Decreased positive affect or pleasure in response to social contacts and usual activities

    c. Social isolation or withdrawal

    d. Disruption in appetite

    e. Disruption in sleep

    f. Psychomotor changes

    g. Irritability

    h. Fatigue or loss of energy

    i. Feelings of worthlessness, hopelessness, or excessive or inappropriate guilt

    j. Recurrent thoughts of death, suicidal ideation, plan or attempt

2. All criteria are met for Dementia of the Alzheimer Type (*DSM-IV*) [7]

3. The symptoms cause clinically significant distress or disruption in functioning

4. The symptoms do not occur exclusively in the course of delirium

5. The symptoms are not due to the direct physiologic effects of a substance

6. The symptoms are not better accounted for by other conditions, such as major depressive disorder, bipolar disorder, bereavement, schizophrenia, schizoaffective disorder, psychosis of Alzheimer disease, anxiety disorders, or substance-related disorders [37]

treatment include suicide plan/threat/attempt, agitation or distress behaviors, implementation of electroconvulsive therapy, self-neglect and/or nutrition risk, and other conditions or living environments that make outpatient treatment inadvisable [37]. Fig 1 provides an algorithm for treatment of mild to moderate depression.

Psychotherapy

Psychotherapy has been shown to be effective as monotherapy or in combination with pharmacologic therapy. Clinical trials have shown that improvement of up to a 50% decrease in depression symptoms has been achieved with psychotherapy and is comparable to outcomes seen with pharmacotherapy [38]. Psychotherapy options include techniques such as cognitive behavioral therapy (CBT), interpersonal psychotherapy (IPT), and psychodynamic therapy (PST). CBT focuses on exploring negative thoughts; IPT focuses on exploring the underlying cause of the depression,

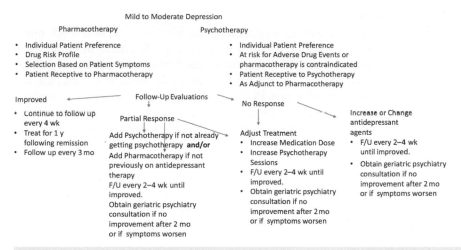

Fig. 1. Treatment of mild to moderate depression.

and PST or "talk therapy" focuses on exploring problems that contribute to depression and finding a solution through an in-depth conversation. Psychotherapy can be used as monotherapy in mild to moderate depression. It should be adjuvant to pharmacologic management in moderate to severe depression and can be effective for patients when pharmacologic therapy is contraindicated. Psychotherapy is typically performed in multiple sessions with 6 to 12 weekly or twice weekly sessions followed by maintenance sessions on a frequency mutually arranged between the PCP and the older adult.

Lifestyle changes

Physical activity has been found to improve symptoms of depression in all age groups. There are multiple pathophysiologic mechanisms of activity that impact mood. It impacts monoamines, thus increasing the availability of serotonin and norepinephrine. Being active impacts cortisol and corticotropin-releasing factor and can reduce the hyperactivity of the hypothalamic-pituitary-adrenal axis, thus decreasing expression of depression symptoms. Clinical studies have shown that 30 to 45 minutes of cardiovascular and strength-building activities per week reduced depression symptoms by 45% compared with 25% of patients in the control group [39]. Older adults with physical disability may have more difficulty with participation in an activity program.

Electroconvulsive therapy

Electroconvulsive therapy is indicated for the treatment of severe major depression. It can be beneficial for older adults who have poor or minimal response to other treatment options as well.

Pharmacotherapy

Pharmacotherapy is a first-line treatment option for management of mild, moderate, and severe depression. There is no significant difference in efficacy between medication classes [40]. Selection of medication class is based on the patient's symptom profile, the side-effect profile of the medication, and the patient's other chronic medications. PCPs should be mindful that efficacy of pharmacotherapy may not be seen for several weeks into treatment. Older adults may take up to 12 weeks, whereas younger populations may see benefit in 4 to 6 weeks.

When prescribing for the older adult, the PCP should follow general geriatric principles of prescribing. The older adult population undergoes physiologic changes related to aging that impact pharmacodynamics and pharmacokinetics that cause drug concentrations and physiologic response to medications less predictable. Slowing and alterations in homeostasis including the following:

- "Start Low Go Slow".
- Change only one medication at a time and anticipate potential interactions are important prescribing guidelines.
- Dosing adjustment with reduced starting doses is required for older adults.
- Review renal dosing adjustment as indicated based on pharmacologic selection [41].
- Consider starting at one-half the usual adult dose and waiting longer for dose increases than with a younger population.
- Evidence has shown that pharmacologic agents have similar efficacy between selective serotonin reuptake inhibitors (SSRIs), serotonin-norepinephrine reuptake inhibitors (SNRIs), tricyclic antidepressants (TCA), and monoamine oxidase inhibitors (MAOIs).
- The safety and side-effect profile of the drug classification impacts selection of pharmacologic therapy for depression (Table 3).

Selective serotonin reuptake inhibitors

SSRIs are considered first line in pharmacologic therapy for depression and are well tolerated in older adults. The main side effect is gastrointestinal upset that is self-limiting and resolved in approximately 2 to 4 weeks after initiation of therapy or dose changes. Citalopram carries a black box warning for potential QT prolongation at higher doses; doses greater than 20 mg daily are contraindicated in older adults.

Serotonin-norepinephrine reuptake inhibitors

The SNRI antidepressants are approved for management of both depression and chronic pain. SNRIs should be considered when the patient has complaints of neuropathic and/or generalized pain with their depression. Side effects of SNRIs include insomnia, nausea, hypertension, and restlessness. SNRIs can cause diastolic hypertension in higher doses. Serotonin syndrome is a condition that manifests with symptoms of tremor, hyperreflexia, fever, confusion, and changes to level of consciousness. Serotonin syndrome can occur with both SSRIs and SNRIs.

Table 3
Antidepressant action and side-effect profile by classification

Drug classification	Drugs in the classification	Mechanism of action	Adverse effects
SSRI	Citalopram Escitalopram Fluoxetine Fluvoxamine Paroxetine Sertraline	Selective inhibition reuptake of serotonin	Gastrointestinal upset Black box warning for potential QT prolongation at higher doses; doses >20 mg daily are contraindicated in the elderly Serotonin syndrome
SNRI	Desvenlafaxine Duloxetine Levomilnacipran Milnacipran Venlafaxine	Selective inhibit reuptake of serotonin and norepinephrine	Insomnia, nausea, hypertension, and restlessness; diastolic hypertension in higher doses Serotonin syndrome
Serotonin modulators	Trazadone	Impact the serotonergic receptors	Sedation Serotonin syndrome
TCA	Amitriptyline Amoxapine Clomipramine Desipramine Doxepin Imipramine Maprotiline Nortriptyline Protriptyline Trimipramine	Inhibit reuptake of serotonin, norepinephrine, and dopamine	Cause or worsen cardiac arrhythmia, confusion, hypotension, narrow angle glaucoma, urinary retention, and constipation
MAOI	Tranylcypromine Phenelzine Selegiline		Hyperadrenergic crisis and serotonin syndrome if dietary and medication restrictions are not followed
Atypical antidepressants	Bupropion	Impact the receptors for norepinephrine and dopamine	Activating effects; contraindicated for patients with seizures or on benzodiazepines
	Mirtazapine	Impact the serotonergic receptors	Increased appetite
Atypical antipsychotics	Quetiapine Aripiprazole	Dopamine and serotonin receptor antagonist	Sedation, extrapyramidal symptoms, weight gain, and elevated blood sugars *Black box warning for increased mortality in the elderly and patients with dementia* Serotonin syndrome

Atypical antidepressants

Mirtazapine and bupropion are classified as atypical antidepressants and are beneficial for older adults with specific symptom presentations with depression. Mirtazapine tends to increase appetite as a side effect and is beneficial for the patient who has decreased appetite or weight loss with their depression. Bupropion works well for patients who have significant lethargy and fatigue because it has stimulating effects; it is contraindicated for patients with seizures or on benzodiazepines.

Serotonin modulators

Trazadone is classified as a serotonin modulator. This medication requires high doses to be effective in the management of depression symptoms and due to this is not used in management of depression. The main side effect is sedation, and low doses are commonly used as a sleep aid.

Tricyclic antidepressants

TCAs are used less often in older adults; this is due mostly to the side-effect and safety profile of this class of drugs. TCAs are highly anticholinergic and may cause or worsen cardiac arrhythmia, confusion, hypotension, narrow angle glaucoma, urinary retention, and constipation.

Monoamine oxidase inhibitors

MAOIs are seldom used because of the dietary and medication restrictions. MAOIs can lead to hyperadrenergic crisis and serotonin syndrome if dietary and medication restrictions are not followed.

Atypical antipsychotics

Quetiapine and Abilify are effective as monotherapy or adjuvant therapy for severe major depression that does not respond fully to other antidepressant medications. Atypical antipsychotics have significant adverse effects, including sedation, and extrapyramidal symptoms. Atypical antipsychotics can contribute to weight gain and elevated blood sugars, which may exacerbate chronic conditions, such as diabetes or heart failure. Atypical antipsychotics also have a black box warning for increased mortality in older adults and patients with dementia.

FOLLOW-UP

Older adult patients with depression require frequent follow-up evaluation. Research has shown that 30% of older adults will not respond to the first-line treatment [37]. Self-discontinuation of medication for depression is seen in 50% of patients in the first 4 weeks of therapy [38]. Patients should be evaluated for medication and therapy compliance, medication side effects, and interactions. Depression scales, such as the PHQ-9 or GDS, should be used to assess for improvement of symptoms, worsening of symptoms, or development of new depression symptoms. Suicidal ideation should be assessed at every visit. Consultation and referral to geriatric psychiatry providers should be considered and offered for all older adults with depression. Older adults with minimal improvement or worsening symptoms, older adults with pervasive suicidal ideation, and those who are intolerant or treatment resistant to psychopharmacotherapy require an interdisciplinary approach, including geriatric psychiatry.

References

[1] Colby S, Ortman JM. The baby boom cohort in the United States: 2012 to 2060: population Estimates and projections. Current population reports. 2014. Available at: https://www.census.gov/prod/2014pubs/p25-1140.pdf. Accessed August 28, 2018.

[2] Hemilick R. Baby boomers retire. 2010. Available at: http://www.pewresearch.org/fact-tank/2010/12/29/baby-boomers-retire/. Accessed August 28, 2018.

[3] United States census bureau an aging nation. Available at: https://www.census.gov/library/visualizations/2017/comm/cb17-ff08_older_americans.html. Accessed August 28, 2018.

[4] Center for Disease Control and Prevention. Health, United States, 2016 with chart book on long-term trends in health. In: DHHS Publication No. 2017-1232. 2017. Available at: https://www.cdc.gov/nchs/data/hus/hus16.pdf#015 2017. Accessed August 28, 2018.

[5] Centers for Medicare and Medicaid. NHE factsheet 2018. Available at: https://www.cms.gov/research-statistics-data-and-systems/statistics-trends-and-reports/national-healthexpenddata/nhe-fact-sheet.html. Accessed August 28, 2018.

[6] Cubanski J. The facts on Medicare spending and financing 2018. Available at: https://www.kff.org/medicare/issue-brief/the-facts-on-medicare-spending-and-financing/. Accessed August 28, 2018.

[7] Gaudette E, Tysinger B, Cassil A, et al. Health and health care of medicare beneficiaries in 2030. Forum Health Econ Policy 2016;18:75–96.

[8] World Health Organization. Mental health of older adults 2017. Available at: http://www.who.int/news-room/fact-sheets/detail/mental-health-of-older-adults. Accessed August 18, 2018.

[9] National Institute of Mental Health. Major depression 2017. Available at: https://www.nimh.nih.gov/health/statistics/major-depression.shtml. Accessed August 18, 2018.

[10] Institute of Medicine. Advising the nation - improving the health 2012 . Available at: http://nationalacademies.org/hmd/~/media/Files/Report%20Files/2012/The-Mental-Health-and-Substance-Use-Workforce-for-Older-Adults/MHSU_olderadults_RB_FINAL.pdf. Accessed August 18, 2018.

[11] van Damme A, Declercq T, Lemey L, et al. Late-life depression: issues for the general practitioner. Int J Gen Med 2018;11:113–20.

[12] Vannoy S, Park M, Maroney MR, et al. The perspective of older men with depression on suicide and its prevention in primary care: implications for primary care engagement strategies. Crisis 2018;4:1–9.

[13] Beyer JL, Johnson KG. Advances in pharmacotherapy of late life depression. Curr Psychiatry Rep 2018;20:34.

[14] Deng Y, McQuoid DR, Potter GG, et al. Predictors of recurrence in remitted late-life depression. Depress Anxiety 2018;35:658–67.

[15] Johannsson O, Lars-Gunnar L, Bjarehed J. 12-month outcome and predictors of recurrence in psychiatric treatment of depression: a retrospective study. Psychiatr Q 2015;86:407–17.

[16] American Psychiatric Association. Diagnostic and statistical manual of mental disorders. 5th edition. Washington, DC: American Psychiatric Association; 2013.

[17] Holvast F, Massoudi B, Oude Voshaar RC, et al. Non-pharmacological treatment for depressed older patients in primary care: a systematic review and meta-analysis. PLoS One 2017;12:e0184666.

[18] Kroenke K, Spitzer RL, Williams JB. The PHQ-9: validity of a brief depression severity measure. J Gen Intern Med 2001;16:606–13. Available at: https://www.ncbi.nlm.nih.gov/pmc/articles/PMC1495268/. Accessed August 28, 2018.

[19] Sheikh JI, Yesavage JA. Geriatric depression scale (GDS). In: Brink TL, editor. Clinical geron-tology: a guide to assessment and intervention. New York: The Haworth Press, Inc; 1986. p. 165–73.

[20] Marak C. Elder orphans: aging without family 2018. Available at: http://www.enlivant.com/blog/elder-orphans-aging-without-family. Accessed August 28, 2018.

[21] Carney MT, Fujiwara J, Emmert BE, et al. Elder orphans hiding in plain sight: a growing vulnerable population. Curr Gerontol Geriatr Res 2016;2016:4723250.

[22] Lixia G, Chun WY, Ong R, et al. Social isolation, loneliness and their relationships with depressive symptoms: a population-based study. PLoS One 2017;12:e0182145.

[23] Miller G. Social neuroscience. Why loneliness is hazardous to your health. Science 2011;331:138–40.

[24] Cacioppo JT, Cacioppo S. The growing problem of loneliness. Lancet 2018;391:426.

[25] National Council on Alcoholism and Drug Dependence [NCADD]. Alcohol, drug dependence and seniors 2015. Available at: https://www.ncadd.org/about-addiction/seniors/alcohol-drugdependence-and-seniors. Accessed August 28, 2018.

[26] Substance Abuse and Mental Health Services Administration [SAMHSA]. Substance use treatment for older adults 2016. Available at: https://www.samhsa.gov/homelessness-programs-resources/hpr-resources/substance-use-treatment-older-adults. Accessed August 28, 2018.

[27] SAMHSA. CAGE AID overview. Available at: https://www.integration.samhsa.gov/images/res/CAGEAID.pdf. Accessed August 28, 2018.

[28] John Hopkins Medicine. CAGE substance abuse screening tool. 2018. Available at: https://www.hopkinsmedicine.org/johns_hopkins_healthcare/downloads/cage%20substance%20screening%20tool.pdf. Accessed August 28, 2018.

[29] Justice in aging. Senior poverty. 2018 Avalable at: http://www.justiceinaging.org/take-action/senior-poverty/. Accessed August 28, 2018.

[30] Choi SK, Meyer IH. LGBT aging: a review of research findings, needs, and policy implications. Los Angeles (CA): The Williams Institute; 2016.

[31] King M, Semlyen J, See Tai S, et al. Mental disorders, suicide, and deliberate self harm in lesbian, gay, and bisexual people: a systematic review of the literature. London: Department of Mental Health, Royal Free and University College of Medicine, University College London; 2009.

[32] Serafin J, Smith GB, Keltz T. Lesbian, gay, bisexual, and transgender (LGBT) elders in nursing homes: it's time to clean out the closet. Geriatr Nurs 2013;34:81–3.

[33] Cavanaugh S, Furlanetto L, Creech S, et al. Medical illness, past depression, and present depression: a predictive triad for in-hospital mortality. Am J Psychiatry 2001;158:43–8.

[34] Polsky D, Doshi J, Marcus S, et al. Long-term risk for depressive symptoms after a medical diagnosis. Arch Intern Med 2015;165:1260–6.

[35] Shaffer D. Physical illness and depression in older adults. In: Williamson GM, Shaffer DR, Parmelee PA, editors. Physical illness and depression in older adults: a handbook of theory, research, and practice. Lawrence (KS): Kluwer Academic Publishers; 2006. p. 22–33; https://doi.org/10.1007/978-0-306-4178-0.

[36] Whooley M, Simon G. Managing depression in medical outpatients. N Engl J Med 2000;343:1942–50.

[37] Teng E, Ringman J, Ross L, et al. Diagnosing depression in Alzheimer disease with the national institute of mental health provisional criteria. Am J Geriatr Psychiatry 2008;16:469–77.

[38] Unutzer J. Late-life depression. N Engl J Med 2007;357:2269–76.

[39] Craft L, Perna F. The benefits of exercise for the clinically depressed. Prim Care Companion J Clin Psychiatry 2004;6:104–11.

[40] Avasthi A, Sandeep G. Clinical practice guidelines for management of depression in elderly. Indian J Psychiatry 2018;60:S341–62.

[41] Shorker A, Hossain MA, Koru-Sengul T, et al. Performance of creatinine clearance equations on the original Cockcroft-Gault population. Clin Nephrol 2006;66:89–97.

Advances in Family Practice Nursing 1 (2019) 33–59

ADVANCES IN FAMILY PRACTICE NURSING

Travel Health for Older Adults

Cynthia Gerstenlauer, ANP-BC, GCNS-BC, CDE, CCD*

Troy Internal Medicine, Troy, MI, USA

Keywords
- International travel • Older travelers • Travel health • Travel vaccines
- Pretravel risk

Key points

- International travel is increasing globally.
- Older adults represent a substantial portion of international travelers.
- Older travelers have special considerations and unique challenges
- Travel medicine specialists are not always available, and primary care providers (PCPs) are increasingly called on to provide pretravel consultation.
- Travel medicine has its own unique body of knowledge and practice guidelines and it is important for PCPs to gain expertise in providing pretravel health.

INTRODUCTION

Globally, there has been a rapid growth in international travel, especially for tourism. Travel from the United States to overseas and Mexico increased from 37 million in 2008 to 66 million in 2016, with destinations to Mexico (38.9%), Europe (17%), the Caribbean (9.8%), Asia (6.7%), Central America (3.7%), Middle East (2.7%), South America (2.5%), and Africa (0.5%) [1]. Older adults represent a substantial proportion of international travelers, with about 30% being aged 60 years or older [2]. This is caused by the increase in the aging population and life expectancy, having the desire to travel, and adequate resources. As travel to emerging economies is increasing, travelers, including those with chronic and active medical problems, are undertaking more adventurous itineraries [3]. Older travelers have special considerations and unique challenges that are important to address in preventing travel-related illness.

Ms C. Gerstenlauer has no commercial or financial conflicts of interest or funding source.

*4600 Investment Drive, Troy, MI 48098. E-mail address: cgerstenlauer@comcast.net

https://doi.org/10.1016/j.yfpn.2018.12.001
2589-420X/19/© 2018 Elsevier Inc. All rights reserved.

As international travel increases, many health care providers from a wide range of disciplines are being asked to provide pretravel advice [3]. Unfortunately, many health care providers may not be trained to meet these needs [3]. A World Wide Web–based survey was done to assess the extent to which primary care providers (PCPs) provided travel medicine advice, and how their understanding and delivery of itinerary-specific advice and management compared with that of travel medicine specialists (TMS) [3]. Of the PCPs, 73% of respondents personally provided pretravel advice, 69% were aware of TMS in their area and estimated that they referred 22% of their patients to them [3]. The top 10 reasons provided for referrals were [3]:

- Lack of travel vaccines in their office
- Need for yellow fever vaccine
- Complex itineraries
- Medical comorbidities
- Pregnancy
- Special purpose of travel
- Children
- Elderly
- Lack of insurance
- Need for malaria chemoprophylaxis

The comfort level with Japanese encephalitis and yellow fever vaccines was greater among TMS. Familiarity with all vaccines increased with volume of travelers and years served in practice. Eighty-seven percent of the PCPs were interested in attending a short course on travel medicine [3].

An airport-based survey of US travelers to low- or low-middle income countries revealed that 46% of these travelers did not seek health information before travel, largely because of a lack of concern about travel health [4]. For those who did, the Internet was the most common source, followed by PCPs; less than a third visited a TMS [4].

TRAVEL MEDICINE

Travel medicine is a young interdisciplinary specialty that has grown into a well-respected discipline with its own professional association, the International Society of Travel Medicine (ISTM) [3]. ISTM has its own body of knowledge, practice guidelines, and Certificate in Travel Health. TMS have in-depth knowledge of immunizations, risks associated with specific destinations, and the implications of traveling with underlying conditions [2]. Most US physicians who provide travel medicine services have training in infectious diseases, internal medicine, or family practice [3]. Nurses play significant roles, being the sole providers of travel advice 22% of the time [3].

A comprehensive consultation with a TMS is indicated for any traveler with a complicated health history, special risks (eg, traveling at high altitudes or working in refugee camps), or exotic or complicated itineraries. However, TMS are not always readily available in communities. The traveler does not have to be physically present to receive pretravel education, so pretravel consultations are ideally suited to be done remotely to give more travelers access to the information they need [5]. Those PCPs who wish to be TMS are encouraged to take advantage of one of the many travel health educational opportunities available, join the ISTM, attend conferences, and obtain their Certificate in Travel Health.

To provide pretravel consultations, a PCP must be able to impart all the necessary information regarding the health risks prevalent in destination countries and possible health prevention measures. This includes information on immunizations and malaria chemoprophylaxis before travel to tropical destinations. PCPs should first become acquainted with the current epidemiologic situation regarding infectious diseases around the world [6]. This is accomplished by accessing the official World Health Organization (WHO) (www.who.int) or Centers for Disease Control and Prevention (CDC) (www.cdc.gov/travel) Web sites. PCPs can also subscribe to a dedicated travel medicine software database designed for TMS to quickly and easily communicate talking points about vaccines, diseases, recent outbreaks, and safety concerns for country-specific destinations, and provide educational handouts for the travelers. Patient handouts are important because the topics tend to be new and the traveler can get overwhelmed. It is important the PCP provide supplemental information that can be reviewed later. Software does not replace travel medicine training or membership in professional organizations, such as the ISTM, but it does help the PCP to provide excellent travel medicine care within the workflow of the office. Authoritative sources, such as Tropimed (www.tropimed.com) and Shoreland Travax (www.travax.com), are in a format that can be used while seeing patients.

THE PRETRAVEL CONSULTATION

Travel health is based on the concept of the reduction of risk [2]. "Risk" refers to the possibility of harm during a planned trip. The pretravel consultation is an opportunity to educate the traveler about health risks at the destination and how to manage them. Attention must be paid to the health background of the traveler, and then incorporate the itinerary, trip duration, travel purpose, and planned activities, all of which determine health risks. Travel health advice should be personalized, highlighting the likely exposures and reminding the traveler of ubiquitous risks, such as injury, foodborne and waterborne infections, vectorborne disease, respiratory tract infections, and bloodborne and sexually transmitted infections. Table 1 outlines the recommended components of a pretravel consultation.

Travelers who are higher risk are recommended to have a pretravel medical check-up to assess their fitness to travel. A typical travel consultation does not include a physical examination, so, a separate appointment with the same or a different provider may be necessary. Travelers with specialized or chronic illness are recommended to see their respective specialists to ensure the best possible disease control.

Table 1
Risk assessment during pretravel consultation

Health Background		
Past medical history	Age	
	Gender	
	Underlying conditions	
	Allergies (especially any pertaining to vaccines, gelatin, eggs, latex, reactions to previous vaccines)	
	Medications	
Special conditions	Disability or handicap	
	Immunocompromising conditions or medications	
	Older age	
	Psychiatric condition	
	Seizure disorder	
	Recent surgery	
	Recent cardiopulmonary event	
	Recent cerebrovascular event	
	History of Guillain-Barré syndrome	
Immunization history	Routine vaccines	
	Travel vaccines	
Prior travel experience	Where has traveled internationally	
	Travel-related illnesses, injuries	
	Experience with altitude	
	Experience with antimalarials	
Trip details		
Itinerary	Countries and specific regions, including order of countries if >1 country	
	Major cities, usual tourist areas vs smaller cities, rural areas, villages	
Timing	Trip duration	
	Departure and return dates	
	Season of travel	
	Time to departure	
Reason for travel	Tourism	
	Business	
	Professional	
	Visiting friends and relatives	
	Volunteer, missionary, or humanitarian relief work	
	Student abroad	
	Adventure (mountain climbing, trekking)	
	Jungle or desert expeditions	
	Pilgrimage	
	Medical tourism	
Travel style	Group or package tour	
	Propensity for "adventurous" eating	
	Traveler risk tolerance	
	General hygiene standards at destination	
	Modes of transportation	
	Accommodations (tourist or luxury hotel, guest house, hostel or budget hotel, dormitory, host family, tent)	

Special activities	Disaster relief
	Providing medical or dental care
	High altitude
	Scuba diving
	Cruise ship
	Rafting or other water exposure
	Cycling
	Extreme sports
	Spelunking
	Anticipated interactions with animals

From Centers for Disease Control and Prevention. CDC Yellow Book 2018 health information for international travel. Atlanta (GA): Oxford University; 2018. Available at: https://wwwnc.cdc.gov/travel/page/yellowbook-home.

Attention to the cost of recommended interventions is important. Travelers must often pay out of pocket for pretravel care, because many health insurance plans do not cover travel immunizations or prophylaxis. Travelers with limited budgets may be at higher risk for travel-associated infections, because they often visit remote areas, stay in lower-grade accommodations, and are more likely to eat local street food [5]. Prioritizing immunizations and prophylactic medications should be part of an individualized assessment based on the travel itinerary, efficacy and safety of vaccines and medications, and associated costs. The traveler may be able to get some vaccines at a lower cost at a health department.

IMMUNIZATIONS

The PCP needs to inform the traveler of the necessity to receive routine and booster doses in line with the vaccination schedule and receive all the required doses of mandatory or recommended vaccinations, with a written confirmation of the doses taken on the International Certificate of Vaccination or Prophylaxis (ICVP or "yellow card") [6]. Preferably, all vaccinations should be taken 4 to 6 weeks before the planned departure, so that there is enough time to receive all doses of the vaccine and develop immunity [6]. Some travelers may be immune to the disease for which immunization is being considered. Testing for antibody titers may be covered by insurance when vaccines are not. Testing for immunity to diseases, such as measles, varicella, and hepatitis A and B, can help determine whether vaccination is required.

ROUTINE VACCINES

All travelers should be current with routine vaccines before international travel, regardless of destination. The benefits of vaccines extend beyond the travel period, and in many cases, lifelong immunity is achieved. A visit to a provider for travel-related immunizations should be an opportunity to bring an incompletely vaccinated person up-to-date on his or her routine vaccinations. Recommendations for the use of vaccines in the United States are developed by the Advisory Committee on Immunization Practices (ACIP) and are published annually. Clinicians should obtain the most current schedules from the CDC Vaccines and Immunization Web site (www.cdc.gov/vaccines/schedules) [7]. Routine vaccines for older adults are found in Tables 2 and 3. For specific vaccines and toxoids, additional details on background, adverse reactions, precautions, and contraindications, refer to the respective ACIP recommendations [7].

REQUIRED VACCINES

There are only a few required vaccines, which need to be prioritized because the traveler may be denied entry to the country without proof of vaccination [5]. Saudi Arabia requires travelers from the United States to have the quadrivalent meningococcal vaccine in the past 3 years, and at least 10 or more days in advance of arrival, for traveling to Mecca during the Hajj and Umrah pilgrimages [9].

Vaccination against yellow fever (YF-VAX) is mandatory for all travelers to several different countries around the world. The yellow fever virus is found in tropical and subtropical areas of Africa and South America. Foreign visitors may be required to present the ICVP/yellow card, documenting the dose they had received before entering some countries, at least 10 or more days in advance of arrival. Be aware that travelers who may be staying in a yellow-fever endemic country only briefly (such as during an airport layover) may still need evidence of vaccination to enter other countries on their itinerary [9]. Since July 2016, when the WHO announced new vaccination requirements for yellow fever, booster doses of YF-VAX are no longer recommended after 10 years for most travelers, because a single dose of YF-VAX provides long-lasting protection [15]. For information about which countries require YF-VAX for entry and which countries the CDC recommends YF-VAX, visit the CDC Travelers' Health Web site (www.cdc.gov/travel). YF-VAX is available only in certified yellow fever vaccination clinics. To locate a clinic, go to https://wwwnc.cdc.gov/travel/yellow-fever-vaccination-clinics/search. To become a YF-VAX center, contact the CDC at yellowfever@cdc.gov to find out who you should speak to at your state health department for more information on becoming certified. Serious reactions to the YF-VAX may occur in any age group, with an overall estimated relative risk of any serious adverse event of 3.8 per 100,000 doses [9]. Travelers older than 60 have a 1.7 times higher risk for a serious adverse event (6.5 per 100,000 doses), and those older than 70 years have a 2.7 times higher risk (relative risk for serious events, 10.3 per 100,000 doses) [9]. If YF-VAX is medically contraindicated, and travel is unavoidable to a yellow fever endemic area, inform the traveler of the risk of yellow fever, recommend mosquito avoidance, and provide the traveler with a vaccination medical waiver. Travelers should be cautioned that vaccination waiver documents might not be accepted by some countries and refusal of entry or quarantine up to 6 days is possible [5].

In February 2017, the WHO recommended long-term travelers staying more than 4 weeks in polio-infected countries (Afghanistan, Laos, Nigeria,

Table 2
Routine older adult vaccines available, influenza vaccines

Vaccine	Trade name (manufacturer)	Age Years	Dose/route	Characteristics
Influenza inactivated vaccines, quadrivalent IIV4	Fluzone ID (Sanofi Pasteur)	18–64	0.1 mL single-dose prefilled, ID	Standard dose IIVs contain 15 μg of each vaccine HA antigen (60 μg for quadrivalents) per 0.5-mL dose
Inactivated influenza vaccines, trivalent IIV3s), standard dose	Afluria (Seqirus)	18–64	0.5 mL prefilled syringe or multidose vial by jet injector, IM	Standard dose IIVs contain 15 μg of each vaccine HA antigen (45 μg for trivalent) per 0.5-mL dose Multidose vials contain mercury (from thimerosal), single doses are preservative free
Inactivated influenza vaccines, trivalent IIV3s), standard dose	Fluvirin (Seqirus)	≥4	0.5 mL prefilled syringe, IM or 0.5 mL from multidose vial, IM	Standard dose IIVs contain 15 μg of each vaccine HA antigen (45 μg for trivalent) per 0.5-mL dose Prefilled syringe contains latex Multidose vials contain mercury (from thimerosal), single doses are preservative free
Adjuvanted inactivated influenza vaccine, trivalent (aIIV3), standard dose	Fluad (Seqirus)	≥65	0.5 mL prefilled syringe, IM	Prefilled syringe contains latex 63% more effective than regular-dose unadjuvanted flu shots
Inactivated influenza vaccine, trivalent (IIV3), high dose	Fluzone High Dose (Sanofi Pasteur)	≥65	0.5 mL prefilled syringe, IM	24% more effective than standard-dose vaccine in prevention of influenza-related events; contains 4 times the amount of antigen, associated with a stronger immune response following vaccination (higher antibody production)

(continued on next page)

Table 2
(continued)

Vaccine	Trade name (manufacturer)	Age Years	Dose/route	Characteristics
Recombinant influenza vaccine, quadrivalent (RIV4)	Flublok (A) (Protein Sciences)	≥18	0.5 mL prefilled syringe, IM	Identical to IIV4 without egg proteins, formaldehyde, thimerosal, antibiotics, latex, gelatin, or preservatives. Contains 60 μg of each antigen that has been associated with greater immunogenicity and 40% improved efficacy than that of vaccines with the standard dose of 15 μg

Abbreviations: HA, hemagglutinin; ID, intradermal; IM, intramuscularly.

One influenza vaccine is given annually, no booster dose recommended.

All influenza vaccines are contraindicated with h/o severe allergic reactions to any component of the vaccine or after previous dose of any influenza vaccine.

Precautions with moderate-to-severe acute illness with or without fever, with history of Guillain Barré syndrome within 6 wk of receipt of influenza vaccine.

People with egg allergies can receive any licensed, recommended age-appropriate influenza vaccine and no longer must be monitored for 30 minutes after receiving the vaccine. An egg allergy other than hives (eg, angioedema, respiratory distress, lightheadedness, or recurrent emesis; or required epinephrine or another emergency medical intervention), IIV may be administered in an inpatient or outpatient medical setting and under the supervision of a health care provider who is able to recognize and manage severe allergic conditions [8].

Data from Refs.[8–12].

Table 3
Routine older adults' vaccines, other than influenza

Vaccine	Trade name (manufacturer)	Age (y)	Dose/route	Schedule	Booster	Indications	Contraindications	Cautions
Herpes shingles vaccine RZV Recombinant adjuvanted	Shingrix (Pfizer)	≥50	0.5 mL, IM	0, 2–6 mo	None	Prevention of herpes shingles; preferred, even if had ZVL shingles vaccine before	Hypersensitivity to drug/class/components	Immunocompromised Acute illness
Herpes shingles ZVL Live, attenuated	Zostavax (Merck)	≥60	0.5 mL SC	Once	None	Prevention of herpes shingles	As above and severe immunocompromised Hypersensitivity to gelatin, anaphylactic to neomycin Tuberculosis, untreated	HIV infection, asymptomatic Acute illness
Pneumococcal PCV 13 13-valent Inactivated conjugate	Prevnar 13 (Pfizer)	19-64	0.5 mL, IM	Once	Every 5 y	Weakened immune system, HIV, kidney disease, asplenia	Hypersensitivity to drug/class/components Hypersensitivity to diphtheria toxoid	Immunocompromised Acute illness
		≥65		Once	None	Prevention of pneumonia and invasive disease caused by *Streptococcus pneumoniae*		
Pneumococcal PPSV23 23-valent polysaccharide Inactivated	Pneumovax 23 (Merck & Co, Inc)	19-64	0.5 mL IM	None	Second dose if received a first dose age <65 at least 5 y ago	Weakened immune system, HIV, kidney disease, asplenia, chronic lung, liver disease, diabetes, alcoholism, smoke cigarettes	Hypersensitivity to drug/class/components	Immunocompromised Acute illness Chronic CSF leakage
		≥65				Prevention of pneumococcal disease, which is any type of infection caused by *S pneumoniae* bacteria		

(continued on next page)

Table 3
(continued)

Vaccine	Trade name (manufacturer)	Age (y)	Dose/ route	Schedule	Booster	Indications	Contraindications	Cautions
Tdap or Td	Td	≥19	0.5 mL IM	10 y	For a tetanus-prone wound, the minimum interval after a previous dose of any tetanus-containing vaccine is 5 y	1 dose of Tdap if did not get it as a child or adult regardless of the interval since the last dose of Td	Hypersensitivity to drug/class/ components Encephalopathy (eg, coma, decreased LOC, prolonged seizures) not attributable to another identifiable cause within 7 d of any previous dose of tetanus	None

Abbreviations: CSF, cerebrospinal fluid; HIV, human immunodeficiency virus; IM, intramuscularly; LOC, level of consciousness; SC, subcutaneously.
Data from Refs.[9,13,14].

and Pakistan) may be required to show proof of polio vaccination on an ICVP when leaving these countries [16].

RECOMMENDED VACCINES

Recommendations for specific vaccines related to travel depend on the time until departure; itinerary; risk of disease at destination; effectiveness and safety of the vaccine; likelihood of repeat travel; duration of travel; and host factors, such as age and other individual characteristics. Recommendations for travelers are not always the same as routine recommendations. For example, most adults born after 1956 are recommended to receive one dose of mumps-measles-rubella vaccine; however, international travelers of this age are recommended to receive two doses [5]. Table 4 presents recommendations for the use, number of doses, dose intervals, indications, precautions, and contraindications for vaccines that may be indicated for travel. When considering rabies vaccine, consider the risk of animal exposure, access to local health care, and availability of rabies immune globulin and rabies vaccine at the traveler's destination. Travelers who decline preexposure immunization should have a plan of action if an exposure occurs. In up to 37% of locations worldwide, rabies vaccine or immune globulin are available only sometimes or never [5]. Review the itinerary in detail to determine the need for Japanese encephalitis vaccine. Some travelers may be able to obtain vaccine at lower cost outside the United States.

MALARIA

The risk of acquiring malaria varies widely, depending on destination, accommodations, and activities during travel. Every pretravel consultation should include detailed advice about preventing mosquito bites. Malarial chemoprophylaxis, if needed, should be offered based on the risk profile of the traveler and possible financial burden. The CDC and WHO recommend that travelers to malarial endemic areas should use one of the available drug regimens listed in Table 5. The table also includes recommendations for self-treatment of symptoms, should a traveler decline chemoprophylaxis. Travelers who raise the question of purchasing antimalarial drugs at their destination must be advised about the risk of inappropriate, substandard, and counterfeit medications and discouraged from this practice [5].

CHRONIC ILLNESSES

Although traveling abroad is relaxing and rewarding, the physical demands of travel are stressful, particularly for travelers with underlying chronic illnesses. Older travelers are more likely to have a chronic illness requiring medication, which can add to potential health problems and complicate prophylaxis for travel-related diseases, such as travelers' diarrhea and malaria [2]. With adequate preparation, travelers with chronic illness can have safe and enjoyable trips, and travel without restrictions. General recommendations for patients with chronic illnesses are found in Box 1.

Table 4
Travel-related vaccines

Vaccine	Trade name (manufacturer)	Age (y)	Dose/route	Schedule	Booster	Indications	Contraindications	Precautions
Cholera CVD 103-HgR vaccine Live, attenuated	Vaxchora (PaxVax, Inc)	18–64	100 mL oral (reconstituted)	1 dose	Undetermined	Traveling to endemic or epidemic regions with active transmission of toxigenic cholera at least 10 d before travel; risk extremely rare, not routinely recommended; more common in VFR and those performing humanitarian aid work in outbreak settings	Hypersensitivity to drug/class/ components	Immunocompromised or close contact

Hepatitis A vaccine inactivated	Havrix (Glaxo SmithKline)	≥19	1 mL IM	Primary 0, 6–12 mo	None	Travel to countries with high or intermediate hepatitis A endemicity	Hypersensitivity to drug/class/components Hypersensitive to neomycin	Hypersensitivity to latex
	Vaqta (Merck & Co, Inc)	≥19	1 mL IM	0, 6–18 mo	None	Postexposure prophylaxis Lack a risk factor but want protection Recommended for chronic liver disease May be recommended to get for weakened immune system, HIV, kidney disease, asplenia, heart disease, chronic lung and liver disease, alcoholism, diabetes		Hypersensitivity to latex

(continued on next page)

Table 4
(continued)

Vaccine	Trade name (manufacturer)	Age (y)	Dose/route	Schedule	Booster	Indications	Contraindications	Precautions
Hepatitis B vaccine	Engerix-B (Glaxo SmithKline)	≥20	1 mL IM	Primary 0, 1, 6 mo Accelerated 0, 1, 2 mo	None 12 mo	Medical care workers; traveling to areas endemic for HBV; behavioral high-risk factors (IV drug users, multiple sex partners, tattooing or acupuncture, expatriates, missionaries, long-term development workers)	Hypersensitivity to drug/class/components Hypersensitivity to yeast	Hypersensitivity to latex Immunocompromised Acute illness
	Recombivax HB (Merck & Co, Inc)	≥20	1 mL IM	Primary 0, 1, 6 mo	None		Hypersensitivity to drug/class/components Hypersensitivity to yeast	Hypersensitivity to latex Acute illness
	Heplisav-B (recombinant) adjuvanted (Glaxo SmithKline)	≥18	0.5 mL single dose vials, IM	0, 1 mo	None	As above Higher levels of seroprotection with fewer doses	Same as above	Immunocompromised Acute illness

Vaccine	Brand (manufacturer)	Age	Dose/Route	Primary	Booster	Indications	Precautions	Contraindications
Combined hepatitis A and B vaccine HepA-HepB	Twinrix (Glaxo SmithKline)	≥18	1 mL IM	Primary 0, 1, 6 mo Accelerated 0, 7, 21–30 d	None	As above	Same as above	Hypersensitivity to latex
Japanese encephalitis vaccine inactivated	Ixiaro (Valneva)	18–65 ≥66	0.5 mL IM	0, 7 d 0, 28 d	12 mo >1 y after primary series	Travel to areas of risk with rural exposure >4 wk or prolonged residence;	Hypersensitivity to drug/class/ components Hypersensitivity to protamine sulfate	Immunocompromised Acute illness Hypersensitivity to protamine sulfate
Meningococcal polysaccharide diphtheria toxoid conjugate vaccine (MenACWY-D)	Menactra (Sanofi Pasteur)	2–55	0.5 mL IM	1 dose	If at continued risk	Required for Hajj Pilgrimage to Saudi Arabia; preferred for whom multiple doses are anticipated (eg, asplenia, microbiologist) Prolonged exposure to local populations in endemic or epidemic areas	Hypersensitivity to drug/ class/components	Immunocompromised Moderate or acute illness with or without fever
Meningococcal Oligosaccharide CRM 197 conjugate vaccine (MenACWY-CRM)	Menveo (Glaxo SmithKline)	2–55	0.5 mL IM	1 dose	If at continued risk		Hypersensitivity to drug/class/ components	Immunocompromised Acute illness

(continued on next page)

Table 4 (continued)

Vaccine	Trade name (manufacturer)	Age (y)	Dose/route	Schedule	Booster	Indications	Contraindications	Precautions
Polio vaccine inactivated IPV	Ipol (Sanofi Pasteur)	≥18	0.5 mL SC or IM	1 dose if has completed a primary series	None	May be needed for long-term travelers to polio-affected countries (Afghanistan, Nigeria, Pakistan, Laos)	Hypersensitivity to drug/class/ components	Immunocompromised Acute illness
Rabies (preexposure) inactivated	Imovax HDCV (Sanofi Pasteur) RabAvert PCEC Novartis	All ages	1.0 mL IM	0, 7 d, 21–28 d	Perform serologic testing for antibody level; if has declined to below the acceptable level, boost every 6 mo for continuous exposure or every 24 mo for frequent exposure	Itineraries and activities that place at risk for rabies	Hypersensitivity to 2-phenoxyethanol, formaldehyde, neomycin, streptomycin, polymyxin B Hypersensitivity to drug/class/ components HIV/AIDS Cancer Immunocompromised	Immunocompromised, acute illness, hypersensitivity to neomycin

Vaccine	Trade name	Age	Dose/Route	Doses	Booster	Where recommended	Contraindications	Precautions
Typhoid vaccine inactivated Polysaccharide	Typhim VI (Sanofi Pasteur)	≥2	0.5 mL IM	1 dose	Every 2 y	Where recommended, especially developing countries, endemic in rural areas of tropical countries, VFR increased risk	Hypersensitivity to drug/class/components	Immunocompromised Acute illness
Oral typhoid vaccine Live attenuated bacterial (Ty21a)	Vivotif (Berna Biotech)	>6	Capsule	4 doses on Days 1, 3, 5, 7	Every 5 y	Same as above Refrigerate capsules; administer 1-h ac with a cold or lukewarm drink	Hypersensitivity to drug/class/components Immunocompromised Taking antibiotics, if taking mefloquine, separate doses by 24 h	Acute illness Persistent or severe vomiting
Yellow fever vaccine live	YF-Vax (Sanofi Pasteur)	≥9 mo	0.5 mL SC	1 dose	None unless an individual country only honors for 10 y	As required by individual countries or travel in regions of yellow fever endemicity	Hypersensitivity to drug/class/components Immunocompromised Hypersensitivity to eggs, gelatin, chicken proteins, thymic disease, concomitant XRT	In persons ≥60 y Acute illness HIV infection, asymptomatic

Abbreviations: HBV, hepatitis B virus; HIV, human immunodeficiency virus; IM, intramuscularly; IV, intravenous; SC, subcutaneously; VFR, visiting friend and relative.

Table 5
Antimalarial drugs for chemoprophylaxis and self-treatment

Generic/Trade name (manufacturer)	Adult dosing	Advantages	Disadvantages
Drugs for chemoprophylaxis Atovaquone/proguanil Malarone (GlaxoSmithKline)	1 tablet 250 mg/100 mg once daily, 1–2 d before arriving in the malarial area, daily while there, and 7 d after leaving the malarial area	Efficacy (>95% for *Plasmodium falciparum* and *Plasmodium vivax*) Shortest period of time to take No known resistance Safety Minor side effects Few drug interactions No photosensitivity Good for last minute travelers Good choice for shorter trips	Take with a meal or milky fluid Side effects: mild headache, GI complaints Should not be used with severe renal impairment (clearance <30 mL/min) Interactions (rifampin, tetracycline, and metoclopramide) Dose of oral anticoagulant may need to be reduced or monitoring of PT may need to be more frequent while taking Cost
Chloroquine phosphate Aralen and generic (Abbott Laboratories)	1 tablet 500 mg once weekly, 1–2 wk before travel in the malarial endemic area, weekly throughout the stay, and 4 wk after travel	Efficacy (in regions with no resistance) Safety Weekly administration Cost Minor side effects Few interactions Good choice for long trips	Use limited by widespread *P falciparum* resistance (all malarious areas except Central America west of the Panama Canal Zone, Mexico, Haiti, the Dominican Republic, and most of the Middle East) Must use IM (not ID) route for rabies vaccination May exacerbate psoriasis, eczema Lengthy schedule Drug interactions (eg, acetaminophen)

Doxycycline Vibramycin and generic	1 tablet or capsule 100 mg once daily, 1–2 d before arriving in the malarial area, throughout the stay in endemic areas and 28 d after travel	Efficacy (84%–98% for P falciparum) No known resistance Safety Cost Minor side effects Good for last minute travelers If already taking for acne, do not need to take an additional medicine	Daily administration Lengthy schedule Side effects (phototoxicity (<10%), vaginal candidiasis, GI complaints) Multiple interactions (alcohol, anticoagulants, sulfonylureas, phenytoin, carbamazepine, antacids, bismuth) Cannot take simultaneously with oral typhoid vaccine
Mefloquine Larium and generic (Roche)	1 tablet 250 mg once weekly, 1–2 wk before travel in the malarial endemic area, weekly while there, and 4 wk after returning home	Efficacy (>90%) against all Plasmodia sp) Safety (serious adverse reactions are uncommon) Weekly administration Good choice for long trips	Efficacy (P falciparum resistance in South East Asia) Some resistance in China, Amazon region, parts of sub-Saharan Africa Cost Frequent neuropsychiatric side effects and GI complaints Drug interactions (eg, anticonvulsants, β-blockers) Not recommended with cardiac conduction abnormalities Lengthy schedule Contraindications (depression, anxiety, psychosis, seizures)

(continued on next page)

Table 5
(continued)

Generic/Trade name (manufacturer)	Adult dosing	Advantages	Disadvantages
Drug for presumptive self-treatment of malaria			
Atovaquone/proguanil Malarone (GlaxoSmithKline) 250 mg/100 mg	4 tablets once daily (can be divided into 2 doses) for 3 d	Efficacy (>95% for *P falciparum* and *vivax* and for multidrug resistant *P falciparum*) As above	Not for those taking Malarone prophylaxis If cannot be used, the CDC Malaria Hotline (770–488–7788) can provide support
Artemether-lumefantrine Coartem (Novartis) 20 mg/120 ng	A total of 6 tablets over 3 d; initial dose, second dose 8 h later, then 1 dose twice daily for 2 d	Treatment of uncomplicated *P falciparum* malaria infections; not for treatment of severe malaria or prevention	Not for those taking mefloquine prophylaxis Take with food Caution for severe renal or hepatic impairment Personal or family history of QT prolongation Recent MI, CHF, bradycardia, ventricular arrhythmias

Abbreviations: CHF, congestive heart failure; GI, gastrointestinal; ID, intradermal; IM, intramuscularly; MI, myocardial infarction; PT, prothrombin time.
Data from Refs.[5,6,9].

Box 1: Management of chronic illnesses while traveling

- Ensure that any chronic illnesses are well controlled.
- Advise to consider a destination where there is access to care for their condition.
- Advise about packing a health kit (see Box 3).
- Pack prescriptions and medical supplies in their original containers in carry-on luggage.
- Carry a copy of their medication list.
- Ensure the traveler has enough medication for the entire trip, plus extra in case of unexpected delays.
- Because medications should be taken based on elapsed time and not time of day, travelers may need guidance on scheduling when to take medication during and after crossing time zones.
- Advise travelers to check with the US embassy or consulate to clarify medication restrictions in the destination country; some countries do not allow visitors to bring certain medications into the country, especially narcotics and psychotropic medications.
- Educate travelers for any drug interactions. Warfarin may interact with medications prescribed for self-treatment of travelers' diarrhea or malaria chemoprophylaxis. If taking aspirin, cannot take acetazolamide for altitude; may be able to temporarily change to a nonaspirin blood thinner.
- Provide a clinician letter: outline allergies, existing medical conditions, medications prescribed (including generic names), and any equipment required to manage the condition.
- Help travelers devise a health plan: provide instructions for managing minor problems or exacerbations of underlying illnesses; include information about medical facilities available in the destination country.
- Wear a medical alert bracelet or carry medical information on one's person.
- Consider advising the traveler to use a mobile application to track certain chronic illnesses while traveling, such as diabetes.
- Diabetes: accept somewhat higher blood glucose levels during travel days to avoid hypoglycemia. Plan for self-management of dehydration, diabetic foot, and pressure sores; insulin adjustments, check blood glucose every 4 to 6 hours during air travel; discuss changes in insulin regimen or oral agent with diabetes specialist; provide PCP letter stating need for all equipment, including syringes or pen needles, glucose meter, and supplies; keep insulin and all glucose meter supplies in carry-on bag; bring food and supplies needed to manage hypoglycemia during travel; check feet daily for pressure sores.
- Notify the airline in advance if oxygen or other equipment is needed on the plane.
- TSA Cares Helpline (toll-free at 855–787–2227) can also provide information on how to prepare for the airport security screening process with respect to a disability or medical condition.
- Prepare for chronic obstructive pulmonary disease or asthma exacerbations by having lung function testing before travel and consider taking stand-by bronchodilators and steroids.
- Persons with significant cardiac disease should visit their cardiologist before travel and carry with them a copy of their most recent electrocardiogram.

- Suggest supplemental insurance; four types of insurance policies are considered:
  - Trip cancellation in the event of illness
  - Supplemental insurance coverage for medical treatment, reimbursement for cost of medical treatment abroad (most medical insurance policies do not cover health care in other countries); some plans do not cover costs for pre-existing conditions; consider choosing a medical assistance company that allows storage of medical history, so it is accessed worldwide
  - Medical evacuation and repatriation insurance
  - Insurance for rescue operation if including high mountain climbing

From Centers for Disease Control and Prevention. CDC Yellow Book 2018 health information for international travel. Atlanta (GA): Oxford University Press; 2018. Available at: https://wwwnc.cdc.gov/travel/page/yellowbook-home.

ALTERED IMMUNOCOMPETENCE

Immunocompromised travelers make up 1% to 2% of travelers seen in US travel clinics [5]. Altered immunocompetence is caused either by a disease (leukemia, human immunodeficiency virus infection) or by drugs or other therapies (cancer, prolonged high-dose corticosteroids). It can also include such conditions as asplenia and chronic renal and liver disease (including hepatitis C). High-level immunosuppression includes human immunodeficiency virus infection with a CD4 cell count less than 200 cells/µL, receipt of daily corticosteroid therapy with greater than or equal to 20 mg of prednisone or equivalent for greater than or equal to 14 days, primary immunodeficiency disorder, and receipt of cancer chemotherapy [5]. Determination of altered immunocompetence is important because the incidence or severity of some vaccine-preventable diseases is higher in people with altered immunocompetence. These immunocompromised travelers pursue itineraries like immunocompetent travelers, so overall, considerations for vaccine recommendations are the same as other travelers. Inactivated vaccines may be safely administered to a person with altered immunocompetence, although response to such vaccines may be suboptimal [5]. Live vaccines should generally be deferred until immune function has improved. If immune function does not improve, live vaccines are contraindicated. If a traveler cannot tolerate recommended immunizations or prophylaxis, then the PCP should consider counseling them to consider changing the itinerary, altering the activities planned during travel, or deferring the trip. The traveler's specialty care provider may need to be contacted to discuss any concerns, such as with drug interactions or contraindications.

Adults with asplenia have specific vaccination recommendations because of their increased risk for infection by encapsulated bacteria. Therefore, certain vaccines, such as meningococcal B vaccine and pneumococcal polysaccharide vaccines, are recommended specifically for people with altered immunocompetence. Table 6 provides specific vaccines recommended.

Table 6
Functional or anatomic asplenia recommended vaccines

Vaccine	Brand (manufacturer)	Age in years	Schedule	Booster doses
Haemophilus influenzae type b Hib	Hiberix (GlaxoSmithKline)	≥19	Unimmunized 1 dose	None
Conjugate protein Meningococcal conjugate (MenACWY-D)	Menactra	≥2	Preferred; 2 doses separated by ≥2 mo	1 dose every 5 y
	Menveo	≥2	2 doses separated by 2 mo	1 dose every 5 y
	Bexsero[a]	≥10	2 doses 0, 1 mo	None
Meningitis B MenB	Truenba[a]	≥10	3 dose 0, 1–2, 6 mo	
Pneumococcal	Prevnar 13	≥19	Unimmunized 1 dose; if previously received Pneumovax 23, ≥12 mo later	None
Pneumococcal	Pneumovax 23	≥19	1 dose ≥8 wk after Prevnar 13; if previously received Pneumovax 23, ≥5 y later	Every 5 y

[a]Same vaccine must be used for all doses.
Data from Centers for Disease Control and Prevention. CDC Yellow Book 2018 health information for international travel. Atlanta (GA): Oxford University Press: 2018; and Tropimed. Available at: www.tropimed.com. Accessed October 25, 2018. Note: Separate MenACWY-D and Prevnar 13 by 4 weeks if possible.

Travelers with the following situations are not considered significantly immunocompromised and should be prepared as any other traveler:

- Receiving corticosteroids less than 20 mg prednisone
- On inhaled, topical, or injectable steroids
- Have not been on high-dose steroids more than 2 weeks for more than a month (or for 2 weeks if was on for <2 weeks)
- Has not been on chemotherapy for more than 3 months and whose malignancy is in remission
- Has an autoimmune disease, such as lupus, inflammatory bowel disease, or rheumatoid arthritis, that is not being treated with immunosuppressive or immunomodulatory drugs [5].

VISITING FRIENDS AND RELATIVES

A traveler is defined as a visiting friend and relative (VFR) if they are an immigrant, ethnically and racially distinct from the majority population of the country of residence, who returns to his or her home country, to visit friends or relatives [5]. In 2014, a total of 37% of overseas international travelers from the United States listed VFR as a reason for travel [5]. VFRs experience a higher incidence of travel-related infectious diseases, such as malaria, typhoid fever, tuberculosis, hepatitis A, and sexually transmitted diseases, than do other groups of international travelers. There are several potential reasons for this [5]:

- They assume they are immune, but typically their immunity has waned and is no longer protective
- Less than 30% seek pretravel health
- Financial, cultural, and language barriers, and lack of access to clinics
- Lack of trust in the medical system
- Tend to travel to higher risk destinations, have last-minute travel plans, and take longer trips
- May stay in family or friends' homes; live the local lifestyle, which may include a lack of safe food and water; and not use bed nets (are eight times more likely to be diagnosed with malaria than are tourist travelers)

It is important for the PCP to increase awareness of VFR travelers regarding their unique risks for travel-related infections and barriers to travel health services. Travel immunization recommendations and requirements for VFRs are the same as those for US-born travelers. It is important to first try to establish whether the immigrant traveler has had routine immunizations or has a history of specific diseases. Adult travelers, in the absence of documentation of immunizations, may be susceptible. The CDC-supported, "Heading Home Healthy program," (www.HeadingHomeHealthy.org) is focused on reducing travel-related illnesses in VFR travelers. The program contains videos, informational resources, and health tools in multiple languages and was developed to assist not only VFR travelers but also their PCPs [5].

Box 2 gives general precautions during travel; Box 3 gives advice on the contents of a travel health kit.

Box 2: General health precautions during travel

- Acclimatization:
  - Drink at least 3 or 4 L of mineral water or isotonic drinks per day
  - Avoid intense physical activity in the first few days after arrival
- Personal hygiene, appropriate clothing
- Water/food and feeding hygiene
- Risks from traffic accidents
- Effective measures against insect bites
  - Insect repellants with N,N-diethyl-meta-toluamide (DEET), 20% to 40%
  - Mosquito nets
  - Wear long pants, long sleeves
  - Avoid staying outdoors from dusk to dawn, when insects are the most active
  - Air-condition the living space
  - Insect screens are properly installed and tightly fitted
  - Treat clothing with permethrin up to 2 weeks before travel
- Avoid animal bites
  - Consider pre-exposure rabies
  - Avoid contact with animals domesticated (dogs, cats) and wild (foxes, monkeys); never approach, stroke, or feed
  - If bitten or scratched by an animal, wash the wound thoroughly with soap and water and seek medical advice; postexposure vaccination may be necessary
- Prevent foodborne or waterborne infections
  - Regularly wash hands with soap and water or disinfecting gel or tissues if soap and water not available, before every meal, and after using the toilet
  - Drink bottled or boiled water only, carbonated drinks, beer, and wine
  - Avoid drinking water with ice cubes (may be contaminated)
  - Avoid food from street vendors
  - Avoid unpasteurized dairy products
  - Eat only fruits washed and peeled by yourself
  - Avoid uncooked vegetables, meat, and seafood
  - Eat preferably recently cooked and hot-served food
- Protection against altitude sickness in high mountain areas
  - Acclimatization
  - Medications (eg, acetazolamide if no sulfa allergy, or alternatives)
- Avoid tattooing, body piercing, injections with nonsterile needles
- Use condoms if travels include engaging in casual sex
- Avoid walking barefoot in areas where local animals defecate

Data from Refs.[5,6,9].

Box 3: Contents of a travel health kit

- Recommended health prevention products (eg, for malaria, altitude)
- Medications; prescription medicines for chronic conditions; keep in the hand luggage in the original packaging; liquid containers larger than 100 mL (3-oz) must be placed in checked baggage; containers smaller than 100 mL may be carried in the hand luggage, but must be stored in a sealed transparent plastic bag
- List of prescriptions and PCPs orders
- Medical history summary
- Contact information for health care providers, family members
- Dressing material; 4 × 4 gauze pads, band-aids
- Adhesive tape/elastic bandage roll
- Disinfectant (eg, 10% povidone-iodine or 70% alcohol)
- Insect repellent containing 30% to 50% DEET or 20% picaridin
- Permethrin spray for clothes, screens, camping gear, and mosquito nets
- Antidiarrheal medication (Imodium)
- Analgesic/antipyretic (eg, aspirin, acetaminophen, ibuprofen)
- Antihistamine (eg, 1% hydrocortisone cream, oral diphenhydramine)
- Antibiotic
- Antibacterial ointments (eg, 1% bacitracin)
- Eye drops
- Extra pair of glasses or contact lenses
- Sunglasses
- Sunscreen with wide spectrum UVA-UVB block SPF ≥15, resistant to water
- Water purification (eg, iodine-containing water purification tablets, tincture of iodine, various filters or sterilizing devices)

Data from Centers for Disease Control and Prevention. CDC Yellow Book 2018 health information for international travel. Atlanta (GA): Oxford University Press; 2018; and Tropimed. Available at: www.tropimed.com. Accessed October 25, 2018.

SUMMARY

International travel is increasing and PCPs are being increasingly called on to provide pretravel health. The PCP needs to be ready to give professional advice to different groups of travelers, such as VFRs, those with chronic illnesses, allergies, immunodeficiency, cardiovascular or respiratory conditions, and psychological or psychiatric problems. The outcome of a pretravel consultation likely depends on the fundamentals of knowledge, expertise and communication skills of the provider, and the health beliefs of the traveler. The CDC and the ISTM have many resources to assist the PCP to become more proficient at travel health [13]. Older travelers represent a minority of patients in travel clinics, but they are known to be at higher risk for travel-related illnesses or injury [2]. Older travelers should be specifically counseled to reduce their risks by obtaining pretravel health, including additional travel insurance.

References

[1] US Department of Commerce, International Trade Administration, National Travel and Tourism Office. Available at: http://tinet.ita.doc.gov/outreachpages/outbound.general_information.outbound_overview.html. Accessed October 25, 2018.

[2] Gerstenlauer C. Pre-travel health in the older adult. Geriatr Nurs 2017;38:599–601.

[3] Kongelman L, Barnett E, Chen L, et al. Knowledge, attitudes, and practices of US Practitioners who provide pre-travel advice. J Travel Med 2014;21(2):104–14.

[4] LaRocque R, Rao S, Tsibris A, et al. Pre-travel health advice-seeking behavior among US international travelers departing from Boston Logan International Airport. J Travel Med 2010;17:387–91.

[5] Centers for Disease Control and Prevention. CDC Yellow Book 2018 health information for international travel. Atlanta (GA): Oxford University Press; 2018.

[6] Korzeniewski K. Travel medicine in primary health care. Fam Med Prim Care 2017;19(3): 303–8.

[7] Available at: http://www.cdc.gov/vaccines/acip/index.html. Accessed October 25, 2018.

[8] Kroger AT, Duchin J, Vázquez M. In: General best practice guidelines for immunization. Best Practices Guidance of the Advisory Committee on Immunization Practices (ACIP). Available at: www.cdc.gov/vaccines/hcp/acip-recs/general-recs/downloads/general-recs.pdf. Accessed October 25, 2018.

[9] Tropimed. Available at: www.tropimed.com. Accessed October 25, 2018.

[10] Izurieta H, Thadani N, Shay D, et al. Comparative effectiveness of high-dose versus standard-dose influenza vaccines in US residents aged 65 years and older from 2012 to 2013 using Medicare data: a retrospective cohort analysis. Lancet 2015;15:293–300.

[11] Dunkle L, Izikson R, Patriarca P, et al. Efficacy of recombinant influenza vaccine in adults 50 years of age or older. N Engl J Med 2018;376(25):2427–36.

[12] Available at: https://www.cdc.gov/flu/about/disease/65over.htm. Accessed October 25, 2018.

[13] Available at: www.cdc.gov/vaccines. Accessed October 25, 2018.

[14] Recommended immunizations for adults by age. 2018. Available at: https://www.cdc.gov/vaccines/schedules. Accessed October 25, 2018.

[15] World Health Organization. New yellow fever vaccination requirements for travelers. Available at: http://www.who.int/ith/updates/20160727/en/. Accessed October 25, 2018.

[16] Available at: https://wwwnc.cdc.gov/travel/news-announcements/polio-guidance-new-requirements. Accessed October 25, 2018.

Advances in Family Practice Nursing 1 (2019) 61–74

ADVANCES IN FAMILY PRACTICE NURSING

ELSEVIER
MOSBY

Ethical Considerations in End-of-Life Care for Older Persons with Lifelong Disabilities

Douglas P. Olsen, PhD, RN[a,b,*], Linda J. Keilman, DNP, GNP-B[c]

[a]Michigan State University, College of Nursing, 1355 Bogue Street, A102 Life Sciences, East Lansing, MI 48824, USA; [b]Sechnov University, Moscow, Russia; [c]Michigan State University, College of Nursing, 1355 Bogue Street, A126 Life Sciences, East Lansing, MI 48824, USA

Keywords

- Older adults • Intellectual disability • Developmental disability • End of life • Ethics
- Justice • Informed consent • Dignity

Key points

- Primary care patients should be as involved as possible in decision making with their known needs and desires accommodated to the extent feasible, even if they lack the decision-making capacity to be fully and legally responsible for the decision.
- Maintaining patient dignity is an ethical priority. Therefore, when considering interventions to control patient behavior, especially medication, it is essential to be self-reflective to avoid bias.
- Ethical decision making is complex and multifactorial.
- Although there are no determinative algorithms for making ethical decisions, an organized rigorous approach identifying and considering all relevant factors is advised.

INTRODUCTION

During the 20th and into the 21st centuries, health care innovations, technological advances, environmental changes, big data, the explosion of genetics/genomics, and pharmaceutical discoveries have led to increased overall aging

Disclosure Statement: D.P. Olsen and L.J. Keilman declare they have no commercial or financial conflicts of interest. No funding sources were used for this work.

*Corresponding author. Michigan State University, College of Nursing, 1355 Bogue Street, A102 Life Sciences, East Lansing, MI 48824. E-mail address: dolsen@msu.edu

https://doi.org/10.1016/j.yfpn.2018.11.002

worldwide. For the United States in 2016, life expectancy by gender was 76.1 years (male) and 81.3 years (female) [1]. This increase in life expectancy describes the general population and also includes individuals living with intellectual and developmental disorders (I/DD). The lifespan for adults with I/DD is currently more than 60 years of age [2]. This longevity trend marks a significant change in the special needs of aging individuals living with I/DD and has a tremendous impact on primary care. Not all health care professionals have been educated to care for this special population into old age. This article seeks to educate primary-care advanced practice registered nurses (APRNs) about aged individuals with I/DD and how to provide ethical, person-centered care as they approach the end of life (EOL) through background information and the presentation of 3 case studies.

BACKGROUND

In the United States, there are 7 to 8 million people (3% of the population) living with some type of I/DD [3]. An intellectual disorder (ID) is characterized by significant limitations in intellectual functioning and adaptive behavior that impacts daily life and social skills [4]. Intellectual functioning is how one thinks, solves problems, reasons, performs activities of daily living independently (bathing, dressing, grooming, oral care, toileting, transferring, walking, climbing stairs, eating), reaches age-appropriate developmental milestones, communicates, retains information, and connects actions to consequences. ID adversely affects educational performance [5]. The range of signs and symptoms can be from mild to profound and is generally diagnosed before the age of 18 years. Risk factors or causes of ID can be genetic, physical, or environmental, but a specific cause often cannot be identified. Down syndrome is the most common genetic origin of ID and results from an extra third chromosome (trisomy 21) [6]. Fragile X syndrome is another genetic condition causing mild to severe ID and is more common in males. ID is associated with limited intellectual capacity and is not the same as mental illness. The more profound the condition, the more comorbid disorders can exist, including autism spectrum disorders, attention deficit/hyperactivity disorder, anxiety disorder, bipolar disorder, depression, impulse control disorder, and even self-injury [7].

Adaptive behaviors are the social, practical, and conceptual skills used every day. These include the ability to follow/obey rules, interpersonal skills, ability to make friends and get along with others, occupational skills, coping skills, sense of personal safety, following a routine or schedule, reading/writing/mathematics, self-esteem, and self-direction [4]. When diagnosing or working with ID individuals, providers must consider their culture, ethnicity, religious/spiritual beliefs, environment, community in which they live and their life goals/values to develop an individualized treatment/management plan. The goal should be that everyone's life story is of value and the plan reflects their individuality.

A DD is a broader category and refers to a group of conditions related to impairments in learning, language, behavior, or physical factors and was defined in the Developmental Disabilities Assistance and Bill of Rights Act in 2000 [8]. A DD generally results from disorders of the developing nervous system. Often called neurodevelopmental disorders, examples include cerebral palsy, epilepsy, and autism. The disorder can occur in utero, early infancy, or during development or brain maturation and generally lasts for the individual's lifespan. DD may include an ID. The APRN should do an evaluation and assessment for a definitive diagnosis on all individuals with suspected symptoms. Causes and risk factors are multifactorial and not always known, but may include genetics, parental health and behaviors (smoking, drinking alcohol), birthing complications, maternal infection during pregnancy, head trauma, and exposure to environmental toxins [9].

I/DD (or IDD) is a general term to convey an ID along with the presence of other disabilities that can be neurologic, sensory, metabolic, or degenerative. The term is vague, and categories can overlap, depending on the information source (foundations, organizations, health care systems, academic institutions, or research) and the purpose (educational services for children, housing options for older adults, community services, support) [10]. In the United States, 30 million individuals are directly affected by an individual diagnosed with I/DD [3].

Families have generally provided the majority of care and housing during formative years and beyond; group homes offer adults the opportunity to live independently with assistance. Longer and healthier lifespans mean that many of these individuals are outliving parents, thus requiring other options for housing. Many times, family members (siblings, aunts, uncles) cannot provide the required level of care in their own homes. Many communities have not kept up with the demand for housing, assistance, support networks, and services needed for the aging I/DD population.

AGING

Heterogeneity increases with age (cognition, function, productivity, quality of life (QoL), and social engagement) and individuals with I/DD experience aging at an earlier age than the general population [11]. Aging for I/DD individuals can start as early as 45 to 55 years of age as compared with 65 to 70 years in the general population [2]. Cognition and function can vary widely among individuals with the same I/DD diagnoses. Individuals with I/DD experience conditions of aging at an accelerated rate, including cataracts, glaucoma, cerumen impaction, osteoporosis, osteoarthritis, gastroesophageal reflux disease, colon cancer, urinary incontinence, and oral health issues [12]. Fall risk increases with age; the early degenerative changes seen in individuals with I/DD puts them at a higher risk for falls [12]. Additionally, individuals with I/DD have unique needs related to their lifelong conditions and earlier aging onset. Some of these issues include:

- Polypharmacy,
- Dental disease,

- Sensory impairment (vision, hearing, taste),
- Dementia,
- Mental illness,
- Functional decline; musculoskeletal issues,
- Obesity,
- Early onset menopause,
- Adult onset seizure disorders,
- Sleep apnea, and
- Cancers [12]

This information is valuable for the APRN, who needs to understand that with accelerated aging, evidence-based guidelines need to be followed that are written specifically for individuals with I/DD. These guidelines take in to consideration the higher risk and need for early screening for conditions that are common in this population. Health promotion/prevention is extremely important in this population to live a fulfilled healthful life.

For those individuals living with parents or other adults in their seventh decade of life and older, the health care needs of both dyads are increasing at the same time, potentially impacting the ability for proper support and care in the home and also speaking to the need for planning transitions of care/housing.

PRIMARY CARE

APRNs in primary care are especially suited to effectively care for older adults with I/DD and help them to self-manage some chronic conditions. Understanding disabilities and comorbid conditions provides a strong foundation for establishing therapeutic working relationships focused on health promotion, disease prevention, protection of human rights, advocacy, and ethical behavior. Using an interprofessional team approach to maximize appointments, care, and information is essential. The coordination and collaboration of care is paramount to optimal access and appointments. Person-centered care should be centered on the self-determination of individuals with I/DD and include communities of support [13].

Inclusivity of care includes asking the older adult what his or her life goals and values are as well as discussions around advance care planning (ACP). ACP would need to involve the individual responsible for making decisions if the older adult lacks capacity, with the goal that decisions are made in the best interest of I/DD individuals and not the patient advocate or guardian. If the older adult can have conversations, discussions should include what they know or understand about growing older and dying and what their thoughts are about their own death. Ideally, these difficult conversations should begin as soon as possible with the adult patient and family members or other designated decision makers. Age should not be the marker for having EOL discussions, particularly when aging is accelerated. In 2014, the Institute of Medicine recommended that ACP begin at any age or any state of health [14]. ACP should be discussed and updated with every visit and treated as a part of the life journey. Appropriately signed documents should be completed and evident in the medical record.

ETHICAL CONSIDERATIONS

Health care professionals are increasingly likely to encounter ethical issues in individuals with I/DD nearing the EOL. Although the form of many of the issues is similar to working with non-I/DD patients, there are substantive variations in the overall presentation, emphasis of ethically relevant aspects, and relationships among stakeholders. Three cases explore and analyze situations related to ethical uncertainty and values conflict that may arise in the care of I/DD patients including surrogate decision making, maintaining dignity under difficult circumstances, and just allocation of resources.

CASE 1: DEVELOPMENTAL DISABILITY AND END-OF-LIFE CARE

Joan is a 69-year-old woman with Down syndrome and mild Alzheimer's disease, as well as other chronic comorbid conditions. Her health has been failing over the last year. Her APRN deems Joan eligible for hospice care and supports this as her best option. Currently, Joan is conversant; that is, she is able to express immediate feelings and needs, such as eating or toileting. However, her orientation to time, place, and situation fluctuates. She has lived in supported housing since age 18, and her 72-year-old sister is her guardian and brings her to her primary care appointments. Joan recognizes her sister about one-half of the time. Lifelong assistance was necessary related to her I/DD needs, including the inability to perform activities of daily living and instrumental activities of daily living (difficulty with finances and planning related to meals and home maintenance). However, Joan maintained supportive employment and had an active social life until her health and cognition became impaired several years ago. Joan is unaware of her prognosis, is a full code, and has no advance care plans or medical orders related to EOL care. Two immediate issues are:

1. Whether to tell Joan about her terminal condition and, if yes, how?
2. Who should make decisions about her EOL care and how?

The initial consideration for both questions is assessment of Joan's mental capacity: Does she have the capacity for EOL decisions and, if not, determining the extent to which her current cognition allows her meaningful participation in directing her life and care.

A primary value in nursing is to encourage patients' control of their care to the extent possible and meaningful. The American Nurses Association Code of Ethics provision 1.4–"The right to self-determination"–declares that, "Patients have the moral and legal right to determine what will be done with their own person." [15] This value is enshrined as the well-known ethical principle of respect for patient autonomy [16].

The chief techniques for enacting patient self-determination by following the principle of respect for patient autonomy are informed consent and advance directives. The requirements for adequate informed consent include:

- Disclosing relevant information,
- Determining patient decisional capacity, and
- Preventing coercive influence to ensure that the patient's decision is made autonomously

ACP is similar, except that the patient is deciding hypothetically about situations that may occur in the future. The decisions in advance directives are made at a time when the same conditions as informed consent apply: patient capacity, adequate knowledge, and lack of coercion. The decisions of advanced directives are somewhat weakened by their hypothetical nature, and the desires expressed in advance directives must be turned into actual decisions often requiring interpretation. One of the most powerful and useful advance directive statements is to name a surrogate decision maker.

In Joan's case, it is not clear if she currently has capacity for making EOL decisions or ever had such capacity. She has no formal advance directive, and the status of any prior statements made about EOL care are unclear because her previous capacity to make such decisions is unknown. Her status under guardianship indicates possible issues with capacity, but on its own does not necessarily mean she lacks capacity for EOL decision making. Guardianship is a legal designation made by a judge based on an inability to independently make certain kinds of decisions in general. A clinical determination of decision-making capacity is decision specific and depends on the complexity of the choices as well as the patient's current mental status.

Joan's decision-making capacity and overall mental status, stability, and well-being should be assessed before deciding whether to discuss the prognosis with her. A discussion of the prognosis would be the first step in involving her in the EOL decision-making process. Withholding the prognosis from a patient is considered unethical because it denies the patient relevant information needed to make further health care decisions. The exception to full immediate disclosure of diagnosis and prognosis is called "therapeutic privilege" and is justified by a determination that the patient's mental state is such that the knowledge would cause disproportionate harm [17]. Patients are told their prognosis to enhance self-determination, allowing them to react to and prepare for imminent death in the manner they choose. Knowledge helps to preserve their dignity and allow them to be an active member of the immediate moral community, rather than keeping their participation passive and dependent on the decisions of others. The choice between conflicting values in Joan's case is between sparing her the pain of knowing about her imminent death or allowing her the opportunity to deal with the ultimate existential reality in her own way.

Persons with moderate Alzheimer's disease can learn, recall, and act appropriately on new information, but may require more effort, skill, and support than patients without an I/DD [12]. If Joan is capable of learning and retaining the knowledge of her demise, she may also be capable of discerning or sensing the situation from the cues of those around her. APRNs would be justified to withhold the prognosis if any of these conditions held:

- Joan could not understand her prognosis,
- Joan could not retain the knowledge, and
- The knowledge would cause Joan excessive harm.

However, if Joan is evaluated as having the mental capacity to retain and react appropriately to information, her dignity would be honored by telling her the prognosis and involving her to the fullest extent possible. If the decision is made to discuss the prognosis with Joan, then she should also be involved in decision making about EOL care to the fullest extent possible without causing undue harm, or giving her sole responsibility over decisions she cannot fully appreciate. Although policy and legal reality require decisional capacity to be regarded as either present or lacking, the phenomena of human understanding does not occur as a yes-or-no determination (Fig. 1), but rather as a continuum.

Therefore, Joan may be assessed as lacking the decision-making capacity to be responsible for making EOL care decisions, such as do not resuscitate, placement on a respirator, based on an inability to understand, appreciate, and reason about the consequences of these decisions while retaining the ability to express reasonable preferences related to the specific procedures. For example, although unable to fully appreciate the consequences of being on a respirator, she may be able to express a preference for mobility and enjoyment of speaking. Her reasonably stated preferences should carry considerable weight when determining treatment.

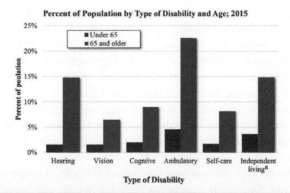

Fig. 1. Percent of the US population in 2015 by type of disability and age. ª Ages 18-64; 65 and older. (*From* United States Census Bureau. Disability characteristics: 2015 American community survey 1-year estimates. 2016. Available at: https://factfinder.census.gov/faces/tableservices/jsf/pages/productview.xhtml?pid=ACS_15_1YR_S1810&prodType=table. Accessed October 25, 2018.)

If Joan is determined to lack decision-making capacity, a surrogate is required to decide and authorize her treatment. The best substitute decision maker is someone who knows her well enough to accurately anticipate her feelings about various treatments and close enough to care deeply about her welfare. APRNs generally do not know the potential surrogates well enough to determine who best expresses these qualities. Further, nurse practitioners should not be arbiters in cases of dispute. Common practice and policy in some institutions identify substitute decision makers by following a hierarchy of relations starting with the individual named by the patient's advance directive followed by guardian, spouse, parent, child, sibling, and so on. For example, the statues regulating policy for the Veterans Health Administration specify an order of priority in individuals sought for surrogate decision making [18].

Following the value of extending self-determination as far as possible, surrogate decision makers should attempt to make decisions consistent with what the patient would have wanted when he or she had capacity. However, in Joan's case, she may not have had decision-making capacity for EOL decisions at any point in her life. If determined that the patient never had such decision-making capacity, the surrogate should make treatment decisions based on an assessment of the patient's best interests. The patient's dispositions and preferences should not go ignored, but be accounted for to the fullest extent possible, considering their feasibility and reflecting the level of appreciation for consequences.

CASE 2: MAINTAINING DIGNITY UNDER DIFFICULT CIRCUMSTANCES

Chester is a 69-year-old man who lived with his mother his entire life. Chester's mother is 95 and recently had a stroke that required hospitalization. Chester was never diagnosed with autism spectrum disorders or attention deficit/hyperactivity disorder, although his psychologist states the patient met the current criteria before his myocardial infarction 5 years ago and was a musical savant when younger. Since the myocardial infarction, Chester's physical and emotional health have declined, and he was diagnosed with vascular dementia. His cognitive state no longer allows him to play musical instruments, and the issue at hand is his failing health and dementia. Chester's threatening behavior and occasional outbursts mean that his siblings cannot care for him, and his mother is scheduled to enter long-term care after discharge from the hospital. Currently, Chester is in a subacute rehabilitation facility after a second myocardial infarction.

Dignity is the central concept leading to the principle of respect for persons. Gallagher states, "Dignity is concerned with the worth and value felt by and bestowed on persons." [19] (p. 591). Like other compelling and essential concepts in ethics, dignity is difficult to define precisely for general agreement. Despite this imprecision, most people recognize the reality of dignity and suggest they can accurately sense its presence and absence. Judgments about dignity are a feature of common speech, although the word may not be invoked,

"She has such poise under these difficult circumstances" or "He belittles the office staff when making routine requests."

Dignity's definition has many variations, but most considerations recognize 2 major aspects: inherent and contingent dignity [19–22]. Inherent dignity is the irreducible worth of all humans. The philosopher Immanuel Kant (1785/1998) said of inherent dignity that it is "not merely a relative worth, that is, a price, but an inner worth, that is, *dignity* . . . humanity insofar as it is capable of morality, is that which alone has dignity" (emphasis in original, p. 42) [23] Inherent dignity is a property of all humans and the same in all humans. Therefore, it cannot be quantified, yet can be recognized or ignored. APRNs recognize patients' dignity or their inherent irreducible worth as human beings, by respecting the autonomy of patients with decision-making capacity and protecting those who hold capacity.

The other aspect of dignity, called contingent or social dignity, depends on circumstances and individual actions [24,25]. Dignity in this sense can be higher or lower. Contingent dignity can also be divided into dignity as felt by the individual and as accorded to the individual by others. Thus, we accord social dignity to an individual who acts selflessly to help others or we perceive loss of dignity in an intoxicated individual acting foolishly. Contingent dignity is not necessarily associated with liability or responsibility. Persons can lose dignity in the eyes of others and themselves through no fault of their own. Think of the patient compelled to disrobe without adequate draping. Unfortunately, the self-perception and, all too often, the public perception of social dignity is unfair. Despite an inability to control or exert personal responsibility for the situation, the poorly covered patient may still feel embarrassment, as do the observers. The detachment of contingent dignity from responsibility creates an obligation to protect vulnerable patients such as the elderly disabled. APRNs protect the social dignity of patients because they value the patient's inherent dignity. Growing older inevitably involves functional losses that put one at risk for loss of social dignity. de Beauvoir (1973) writes, "It is old age, rather than death, that is to be contrasted with life. Old age is life's parody, whereas death transforms life into a destiny" [26] (p. 539). Disability by its nature affects functionality as well as putting the person at particular risk of being perceived as other or different by many in society and therefore with lower social dignity [27,28].

Protection of dignity is difficult in Chester's case. His dignity is at risk from his own behavior and from the treatment used to control the behavior. Further, his behavior can place the safety of others at risk. Exhibiting uncontrolled violent or hostile behavior or sexual acting out diminishes a patient's dignity in the eyes of others as well as in his or her own eyes, if the patient has the capacity to become aware of the behavior and its effects later on. It can be extremely embarrassing to realize that one has behaved badly, especially if another person was hurt physically or emotionally. Therefore, it is an obligation of respect for the patient's dignity to attempt to prevent violent, hostile, or other out-of-control behavior.

Unfortunately, some interventions to curtail such behavior risk, damaging patient dignity. Heavy sedation and physical restraint diminish a patient's social dignity. Psychosocial interventions, such as distraction and de-escalation, which do not involve physical or chemical restriction of the patient's behavior, are ethically preferable to sedation and restraint. In many cases, it is a legal requirement to use the least restrictive method required to ensure safe behavior. Therefore, before using chemical or physical restraints, good faith attempts to use less restrictive measures should be tried and documented.

Interventions like anger management may not be fully applicable in Chester's case, although modified techniques and principles of anger management and other psychosocial strategies may be useful even with persons with diminished capacity. Patients who lack the capacity for treatment decisions should still be involved in their treatment to the degree their ability allows. To aid the patient's involvement, APRNs working with a patient like Chester should use de-escalation and recognize signs of impending behavioral problems. His management plan should identify triggers and include interventions for his behaviors. Unfortunately, behavioral (or nonpharmacologic) interventions do not always work. Medicating a patient to prevent behavioral acting out without overmedicating the patient can be difficult, especially in older adults, owing to metabolic variation and in patients with limited ability to communicate. If Chester lacks the capacity to consent to medication, an appropriate surrogate decision maker should be consulted. The ethical risk is that overmedicating can make the difficult patient much easier for staff to handle. This is a chronic problem in group living situations for older individuals with I/DD. The ability to self-reflect about one's motives in care is an essential skill for ethical practice. Greater awareness can help to decrease the rate of overmedication. For example, antipsychotic prescriptions for older adult patients were reduced simply by sending letters to physicians comparing their prescriptive practices with other prescribers [29].

CASE 3: JUST ALLOCATION OF RESOURCES

Pete is a 72-year-old man with severe autism living in a group home. He has been in monitored group living since age 12. As a child, his outbursts were too difficult for his family to handle at home, and educational resources were not mandated yet by law. He can toilet and feed himself with minimal assistance. He communicates with a series of guttural noises. As he has aged, his behavioral outbursts calmed, and he now lives comfortably and apparently happily with the other residents. However, he continues to have anxiety related to medical and dental procedures, which are conducted with sedation. Fortunately, he takes medication without complaint or difficulty.

As an adult, Pete developed ataxia from an unknown cause. He can move around on his own, but must use his hands to bear weight and steady himself as he navigates around the residence. During his daily walk to the kitchen for breakfast, he stumbled and thrust his right hand through a glass cabinet door, injuring major nerves, tendons, and blood vessels. He underwent emergency repair and was placed in a splint. He awoke terrified in the postanesthesia care unit and attempted to bolt. During the restraint activity, his splint was dislodged and his wound disrupted. His behavior in the hospital was manageable from that point on with round-the-clock sitters that he knew from his residence. He required another surgery followed by extensive rehabilitation to recover enough function in his hand to ambulate in his usual manner. His mother, age 94, is his guardian, but there is some suggestion that she has mild dementia.

The dilemma in this case, given Pete's functioning and the extensive rehabilitation needed, is whether it is more ethical to proceed with or deny him surgery. Two legitimate values are in conflict: First, relying on the principle of beneficence, that is to do what is best for others, APRNs want to help Pete live with the highest QoL possible. The second value is fairness or justice; it might not be fair to use the resources needed for surgery and rehabilitation if the good Pete receives is outweighed by the good others might get from those resources. The risk of a biased perspective of Pete's QoL emerges simply because he has I/DD. His QoL might not be judged fairly because the sources and expressions of his pleasure differ markedly from the typical patient and caution is needed to avoid bias based on Pete's limitations. The APRN who has cared for him in primary care for 20 years is the best candidate to consult on these considerations.

To make this determination, the question that must be answered is, "Under what conditions would it be ethical to forgo surgery with potential benefit?" To begin answering this question, the providers should identify those variables and factors that might influence degree good gained or lost for either Pete or society. These are referred to as ethically relevant variables and in this case include:

- The degree of potential benefit from the surgery,
- The likelihood of Pete gaining the benefit,
- The degree of harm from not doing the surgery,
- The cost of doing the surgery and rehabilitation in money, time, and effort by Pete and others,
- The cost of not doing the surgery, and
- Others' claim to the resources.

Each of these consideration can be examined in Pete's case.

Potential benefit
Pete needs the use of his hands to assist with safe ambulation. Without the surgery, Pete could no longer ambulate independently, significantly diminishing Pete's QoL. Therefore, there is great potential benefit from the surgery.

Likelihood of gaining the benefit
The surgeon is confident that she can repair the tendons, although the success of this procedure depends on a vigorous and protracted rehabilitation program. Because Pete's disability involves cognitive function and he is known to have difficulties with medical procedures, it is legitimate to assess his ability to

tolerate the rehabilitation enough to gain benefit from the surgery. In Pete's case, his APRN and surgeon decide that using familiar carers and approaches could allow his successful completion of rehabilitation. In addition, those who know him best suggest he has a sense of the procedure's purpose and consequences.

Harm from not acting

Pete could not ambulate with the injured hand even after healing, and attempts to use the hand would cause severe pain.

Costs of surgery

The surgery requires a hospital stay of about 5 days and another 3 weeks in a rehabilitation facility for the initial phases of the recovery. The time and effort needed for rehabilitation could be available for others if not used for Pete.

Cost of not doing the surgery

The cost of Pete's care will increase if he is not ambulatory. Further, being non-ambulatory might lead to an earlier death.

Pete's claim to the resources

Members of society have an interest in how pooled resources are used and are involved in decisions of justice in allocating those resources. If Pete were wealthy, for example, and could self-pay the entire cost, society would have a greatly diminished role in determining the appropriateness of doing the procedure. Society might have some interest because it likely contributed to some resources, for example, subsidizing the education of providers. Pete would use Medicare and Medicaid to pay the procedure's costs. As a citizen, he has a legitimate claim to appropriate use of the resources, and society has some claim in determining the appropriateness of the surgery.

Although this suggested algorithm closely follows major ethics principles, the key to the ethical treatment of Pete relies on a moral conception of relationship, that is, avoiding bias about his disability and age in considering the worth and quality of his life. If we eliminate bias about QoL in disability and seniority, the cost benefit calculation of Pete's surgery is similar to that of surgery of other patients.

SUMMARY

These 3 cases do not involve all the potential ethical issues that can arise in EOL care of older adults with I/DD, but are representative of the range and major types of potential issues, including ethical decision making, considerations of the degree of decisional capacity, the proper treatment of 1 patient for the benefit of others, the most ethical ways to involve patients in their own care, maximizing patient dignity, and just allocation of resources. These issues are similar to those for patients who are not disabled, but I/DD is an influential context in which these considerations take place.

Although the principles of ethics play a crucial role in considering these cases, the relational component and context is equally determinative of the ethical perspective. In the first case, APRNs are concerned with the best way to discuss a terminal prognosis with the patient. In the second case, self-reflection is critical for APRNs to ensure that interventions are for the patient's benefit and not to ease the burden of care at the patient's expense. Similarly, in the final case, self-reflection is critical to ensure that bias regarding the patient's disability does not enter into the decision about the just use of resources. Therefore, APRNs must be aware of how a patient's disability influences their experience of disease and the clinician's experience with the patient. More and more individuals with I/DD will be aging in the community and being followed in primary care for their health care needs. The APRN is ideally suited to care for older adults with I/DD in a holistic, person-centered manner. Learning more about older adults with I/DD and reviewing evidence-based guidelines for I/DD patient health care would be prudent as APRNs experience primary care taking on these unique individuals as life-long patients.

References

[1] National Center for Health Statistics. Mortality in the United States, 2016. Available at: https://www.cdc.gov/nchs/data/databriefs/db293.pdf. Accessed October 24, 2018.

[2] Massachusetts Department of Developmental Services. 2014 mortality report. 2017. Available at: http://shriver.umassmed.edu/sites/shriver.umassmed.edu/files/CDDER/QINA%20Aging%20with%20IDD%20finalv2%20tagggged.pdf. Accessed October 25, 2018.

[3] Empower. Intellectual/developmental disability (IDD) fact sheet. Available at: http://empower-wny.org/wp-content/uploads/2016/08/Fact-Sheet-final3.pdf. Accessed October 23, 2018.

[4] American Association on Intellectual and Developmental Disabilities. Intellectual disability. 2018. Available at: http://aaidd.org/intellectual-disability/definition. Accessed October 24, 2018.

[5] National Down Syndrome Society. What is an intellectual disability?. 2018. Available at: https://www.ndss.org/resources/what-is-an-intellectual-disability/. Accessed October 24, 2018.

[6] O'Connor C. Trisomy 21 causes Down syndrome. Nat Educ 2008;1:42. Available at: https://www.nature.com/scitable/topicpage/trisomy-21-causes-down-syndrome-318. Accessed October 25, 2018.

[7] Sulkes SB. Intellectual disability. In: Merck manual professional version. 2018. Available at: https://www.merckmanuals.com/professional/pediatrics/learning-and-developmental-disorders/intellectual-disability#v1105061 2018. Accessed October 24, 2018.

[8] Hahn JE. Minimizing health risks among older adults with intellectual and/or developmental disabilities: clinical considerations to promote quality of life. J Gerontol Nurs 2012;38: 11–7.

[9] Centers for Disease Control and Prevention. Developmental disabilities. 2018. Available at: https://www.cdc.gov/ncbddd/developmentaldisabilities/facts.html. Accessed October 24, 2018.

[10] Eunice Kennedy Shriver National Institute of Child Health and Human Development. Intellectual and development disabilities (IDDs): condition information. 2016. Available at: https://www.nichd.nih.gov/health/topics/idds/conditioninfo/default. Accessed October 23, 2018.

[11] Moran J. Aging and Down syndrome: a health and well-being guidebook. 2013. Available at: http://www.ndss.org/wp-content/uploads/2017/11/Aging-and-Down-Syndrome.pdf. Accessed October 24, 2018.

[12] Tinglin CC. Adults with intellectual and developmental disabilities: a unique population. Today's Geriatric Medicine 2013;6:22.

[13] Heller T. Service and support needs of adults aging with intellectual/developmental disabilities. In: Testimony to the U.S. Senate committee on aging, working and aging with disabilities: from school to retirement. 2017. Available at: https://www.aging.senate.gov/imo/media/doc/SCA_Heller_10_25_17.pdf 2017. Accessed October 24, 2018.

[14] Institute of Medicine. Dying in America: improving quality and honoring individual preferences near the end of life. 2014. Available at: http://www.nationalacademies.org/hmd/~/media/Files/Report%20Files/2014/EOL/Report%20Brief.pdf. Accessed October 24, 2018.

[15] American Nurses Association. Code of ethics for nurses with interpretive statements. 2nd edition. Silver Spring (MD): American Nurses Association; 2015.

[16] Beauchamp TL, Childress JF. Principles of biomedical ethics. 7th edition. New York: Oxford University Press; 2013.

[17] Bostick NA, Sade R, McMahon JW, et al. Report of the American Medical Association Council on Ethical and Judicial Affairs: withholding information from patients: rethinking the propriety of "therapeutic privilege." J Clin Ethics 2006;17(4):302.

[18] 38 CFR 17.32 (a) (iii) Informed consent and advance care planning. Available at: https://www.law.cornell.edu/cfr/text/38/17.32. Accessed October 25, 2018.

[19] Gallagher A. Dignity and respect for dignity – two key health professional values: implications for nursing practice. Nurs Ethics 2004;11(6):587–99.

[20] Lucas K. Workplace dignity: communicating inherent, earned, and remediated dignity. J Manag Stud 2015;52(5):621–46.

[21] Stievano A. Nursing's professional respect as experienced by hospital and community nurses. Nurs Ethics 2016;12:0969733016664972.

[22] Hodson R. Dignity at work. Cambridge (United Kingdom): Cambridge University Press; 2001.

[23] Kant I. Groundwork for the metaphysics of morals. Cambridge (United Kingdom): Cambridge Press; 1998 M. Gregor.

[24] Edlund M, Lindwall L, Post IV, et al. Concept determination of human dignity. Nurs Ethics 2013;20(8):851–60.

[25] Sabatino L, Stievano A, Rocco G, et al. The dignity of the nursing profession: a meta-synthesis of qualitative research. Nurs Ethics 2014;21(6):659–72.

[26] de Beauvoir S. The coming of age. New York: Warner; 1973. P. O'Brian.

[27] Goffman E. Stigma: notes on the management of spoiled identity. New York: Simon & Shuster; 1963.

[28] Staniland L. Public perceptions of disabled people. Evidence from the British social attitudes survey. London: Office of Disability Issues; 2009. Available at: https://www.gov.uk/government/publications/public-perceptions-of-disabled-people-evidence-from-the-british-social-attitudes-survey-2009. Accessed October 24, 2018.

[29] Sacarny A, Agrawal S. Effect of peer comparison letters for high-volume primary care prescribers of quetiapine in older and disabled adults: a randomized clinical trial. JAMA Psychol 2018;75(10):1003–11.

Advances in Family Practice Nursing 1 (2019) 75–86

ADVANCES IN FAMILY PRACTICE NURSING

Improving the Care of Women with Vulvovaginal Atrophy in Primary Care

Susan G. Wiers, DNP, FNP-BC

Wayne State University, 134 Cohn Building, 3555 Cass Avenue, Detroit, MI 48202, USA

Keywords
- Vulvovaginal atrophy • Genitourinary syndrome of menopause • Primary care
- Quality of life

Key points

- Vulvovaginal atrophy is prevalent and burdensome affecting up to 50% of menopausal women having a negative impact on quality of life for women comparable with other chronic conditions.

- Vulvovaginal atrophy is largely unaddressed despite availability of effective treatments because of patient and provider communication barriers, such as embarrassment and lack of knowledge. Safe, effective treatments for vulvovaginal atrophy are available and within the primary care HCPs scope of practice.

- Primary care HCPs should be on the forefront of identifying and treating vulvovaginal atrophy thus improving the quality of life of women.

O lder adults account for nearly 15% of the United States population with this number anticipated to peak at more than 20% when the last of the Baby Boomer generation reaches age 65 in 2029 [1]. It is critical that health care providers (HCPs) make the identification and treatment of common geriatric conditions a priority. One such condition is the genitourinary syndrome of menopause (GSM), which includes the highly prevalent, significantly burdensome, and undertreated genital and lower urinary tract symptoms caused by hypoestrogenism [2,3]. GSM is progressive and affects genital and urinary tract health, sexuality, and quality of life (QOL). Despite the availability of safe, effective therapies for GSM, these symptoms are largely untreated because of patient and provider barriers [4,5]. This article seeks to

E-mail address: gf6140@wayne.edu

https://doi.org/10.1016/j.yfpn.2018.12.002
2589-420X/19/© 2018 Elsevier Inc. All rights reserved.

raise HCP awareness and understanding about the impact and the evaluation and management of genital symptoms caused by vulvovaginal atrophy (VVA) related to natural menopause. Readers interested in urinary symptoms of GSM, specifically urinary incontinence, are referred to a recently published article on the topic [6]. A glossary of common terms is provided in Table 1.

BACKGROUND
Prevalence
GSM is the term approved by the Board of Trustees of the North American Menopause Society and the International Society for the Study of Women's Sexual Health replacing the prior terminology of VVA and atrophic vaginitis [7]. GSM is a group of signs and symptoms resulting from decreased circulating serum levels of estradiol causing vulvovaginal and urinary tract atrophy [2,3]. Quantifying the prevalence of VVA is challenging because of underreporting and variations in study designs; estimates range from 12% to more than 50% rising over time in menopausal women and with high prevalence occurring by the third year of menopause [7–9].

Burden
Bothersome genital tract symptoms occur in up to 50% postmenopausal women with more than half reporting moderate to severe symptoms [10]. Symptoms of VVA include vulvovaginal dryness, burning, pruritis, soreness,

Table 1
Glossary of terms

Term	Definition
Climacteric	Physiologic period associated with termination of ovarian function in menopausal women
Collagen	A polypeptide substance found in mammalian's skin, connective tissue, bone, and teeth
Dyspareunia	Genital pain associated with sexual intercourse
Elastin	Stretchable fibers
Endometrial	Mucous membrane lining of the uterine cavity
Estrogenized	Effects of the interaction of estrogen receptors in target tissues with estrogen compounds
First-pass effect	When an orally administered drug is well-absorbed into the portal circulation but metabolized extensively by the liver before reaching systemic circulation
Hyperplasia	An abnormal increase in the number of tissue cells
Hypoestrogenism	Lower than normal levels of estrogen
Parabasal cells	Vaginal epithelial cells
Phimosis	Intractable foreskin
Postcoital	Following intercourse
Pruritis	Intense itching sensation
Rugae	Ridges produced by folding of an organ wall

Data from Refs.[36–42].

irritation, dyspareunia, delayed or decreased organisms, diminished arousal, and decreased lubrication with sexual activity along with postcoital bleeding and vaginal discharge [2,5,7,10]. Furthermore, VVA is the most common cause of dyspareunia in postmenopausal women [11]. When symptomatic, VVA negatively affects QOL for women and their sexual partners with nearly 60% of women with VVA reporting negative effects on their sex lives [4,5,9,12].

In the United States, severity of genital symptoms related to menopause have been found to be correlated with advancing age, living with a spouse or partner, higher annual household income, and less frequent alcohol use [10]. Worse severity of symptoms correlates with higher comorbidity burden and clinically and statistically significant decreased QOL when controlling for comorbidities and health behaviors [10]. Poor QOL for women with genital tract atrophy has been found to be comparable with those with other chronic health conditions, such as arthritis, chronic obstructive pulmonary disease, asthma, overactive bladder, and irritable bowel syndrome [10]. Whereas climacteric symptoms of hot flashes and night sweats are transient, resolving over time, VVA worsens unless treated [13].

COMMUNICATION BARRIERS

Communication barriers between patients and HCPs hinder initiation of discussion about VVA [14]. Most women with VVA symptoms do not discuss them with their HCPs for many reasons including lack of recognition of symptom attribution to menopause, unawareness of the condition, and assuming their symptoms are normal [8,11,12]. Women may be reluctant to discuss this sensitive topic out of embarrassment and concern that their symptoms would be dismissed by their HCPs [12,14]. Thus, it behooves HCPs to purposefully inquire about VVA symptoms.

Although 40% of participants indicate they anticipated their HCP would initiate discussion about menopausal symptoms, HCPs fail to do so [12]. Kingsberg and colleagues [12] found that 25% of respondents reported seeing any provider in the previous year and, of those who saw an HCP for gynecologic care, only 19% were asked about their sexual health. In the Women's EMPOWER survey, more than 40% of respondents indicated they would have liked to receive written material on vaginal symptoms or would have liked to be given a questionnaire to fill out at the time of their health care appointment; 33% would have liked information mailed to them [15].

Even when women do initiate discussion about their symptoms, many do not receive treatment [14]. HCPs often do not possess adequate knowledge about VVA, are embarrassed to broach topics associated with sexual issues, and express concern about time constraints in a busy practice [12,14]. In women whose HCPs discuss VVA, they have been found to be twice as likely to be current users of medication for their symptoms [12]. Women desire their HCPs to initiate discussion and provide information about VVA and are more likely to get treatment if their HCP inquiries about VVA symptoms and burden. Thus, it is incumbent on HCPs to be proactive by evaluating women for symptoms of VVA, educating women about the progressive nature of and available treatments for VVA, and offering treatment [14].

PATHOPHYSIOLOGY
Premenopausal physiology
The epithelium of the vulva and vagina are estrogen receptor dense tissues [8]. During the reproductive years, endogenous estrogen (predominantly estradiol) effects promote cellular proliferation and maturation maintaining vaginal health [7,8]. Vaginal tissue exposed to estrogen is rich in glycogen, which acts as a substrate for lactobacilli, resulting in an acidic epithelial barrier through production of lactic acid. Acidic epithelium supports bacterial flora, which competitively excludes pathogens through bacteriostatic and bactericidal activity [4,5]. Estrogenized vaginal tissue promotes blood flow, secretions, and epithelial thickness and elasticity allowing expansion and elongation during sexual arousal [5,14].

Menopausal changes
Women are considered menopausal after 12 months of amenorrhea following a final menses [16]. Serum estrogen levels drop off precipitously after menopause [14]. Hypoestrogenism results in reduced genital blood flow, epithelial cytology changes from predominantly superficial and intermediate cellularity to a predominance of parabasal cells, loss of vaginal rugae, and elasticity causing narrowing and shortening of the vagina and may result in strictures and narrowing of the introitus [17]. Loss of superficial epithelial cells with reduced collagen and elastin cause mucosal thinning and decreased vaginal gland secretions resulting in reduced lubrication [5,11]. Additionally, reduced glycogen leads to lower lactobacilli lactic acid production with subsequent loss of the protective properties of an acidic environment resulting in susceptibility to infection caused by pathogens indigenous to the gastrointestinal tract, sexually transmitted infections, and bacterial vaginosis [5]. Connective tissue and smooth muscle of the vulva and vagina are affected by diminished estrogen stimulation. The labia majora can lose subcutaneous fat; the labia minora and clitoris may lose tissue and retract with relative prominence of the urethral meatus rendering it vulnerable to irritation and trauma [5,11]. Additional physiologic changes and symptoms of menopause are listed in Table 2.

DIAGNOSIS
Severity of symptoms does not consistently correlate with physical findings making history and examination essential for diagnosis; in clinical practice, the diagnosis of VVA is primarily made by obtaining a thorough history and clinical examination [4,5]. Non–estrogen deficiency causes for vulvovaginal complaints must be explored [18]. Differential diagnoses include nonmalignant dermatoses, infection, inflammatory conditions, pelvic radiation, prior surgeries, systemic medications, and vaginal or vulvar malignancies [3,4,8,18].

Table 2
Genital symptoms and signs of the genitourinary syndrome of menopause

Location	Symptoms	Signs
Vulva and labia	Dryness, irritation, pain	Loss of fulness
Clitoris	Trauma	Phimosis of clitoris
Vagina	Dyspareunia	Stricture of introitus
	Decreased genital arousal	Vaginal narrowing and
	Pain	shortening
	Burning	Loss of rugae
	Yellow or brown discharge	Both erythema and pallor
	Odor	with a glazed appearance
	Infection	Dry epithelium
	Tears	Brown or yellow secretions
	Petechiae	Petechiae
	Ulcerations	Contact bleeding
		Obliterated fornices with cervix
		flush with vault

Data from Refs.[4,5,11,26,27].

History

All perimenopausal and menopausal women should be screened for VVA symptoms during a routine review of systems [4]. Because of the sensitive nature of VVA and its effects, questions should be carefully worded to minimize patient discomfort [19]. Helpful strategies for uncomfortable conversations include using a direct approach with matter-of-fact open-ended questioning; maintaining eye contact; demonstrating empathy; and ensuring privacy, such as asking third parties to leave the room while questioning [19–21]. Inquiry should include questions about the presence of symptoms (see Table 2) and symptom burden. Information obtained should include onset, duration, severity, any past treatments, and effect on QOL [4]. A sexual history includes the presence of current partners, frequency of sexual activity, and the effect of symptoms on sex life and partner relationships [4]. History should include evaluation for other causes including pelvic radiation, prior surgeries, and systemic medications [8]. Additionally, information should be obtained about prior treatment and efficacy [4].

A subjective appraisal of vaginal atrophy can include establishing the woman's most bothersome symptom at baseline and at subsequent follow-up evaluation [22]. This is done by asking the woman to rate the severity (mild, moderate, or severe) of the symptoms of vaginal dryness, vaginal itching/irritation, and dyspareunia and then asking her which of these three symptoms was most bothersome [22]. Alternatively, Erekson and colleagues [23] developed and tested the 21-item Vulvovaginal Symptoms Questionnaire (VSQ) to measure the presence and effect of symptoms. The VSQ was found to be reliable and have internal consistency with reasonable validity [23]. However, the VSQ might be best suited for women with primarily vulvar (vs vaginal) symptoms [24]. Finally, the Day-to-Day Impact of Vaginal Aging (DIVA) is a 19-item self-administered questionnaire developed to assess the impact of menopausal vaginal symptoms in women of diverse backgrounds and is used for women identified with vaginal symptoms of GSM [24].

Physical assessment

Women with symptoms of VVA warrant a pelvic examination, either at the time of screening or at a dedicated follow-up appointment. External genital visualization of a woman with VVA typically reveals loss of pubic hair, a pale and atrophic vulva with loss of labial and vulvar fullness, and eventual loss of clear differentiation between the labia majora and minora [4,5,25]. Vulvar examination should include evaluation for evidence consistent with other disorders and etiologies including dermatitis (caused by soaps, perfumes, powders, and panty liners), erosive lichen planus, lichen sclerosis, infection, trauma, foreign bodies, and malignancy [4,18]. Urethral prominence in relation to the labia and clitoral atrophy may be noted; the urethral meatus may be everted with a distended and/or red appearance and should be examined for possible trauma [4,5].

Vaginal examination with a speculum may be difficult or impossible because of shortening of the vagina and narrowing of the introitus. Use of a lubricated pediatric speculum may be helpful [4]. The vagina should be evaluated for injury and loss of integrity, such as vaginal tears, lacerations, and ulcerations [8]. Vaginal pH point-of-care testing is done with a cotton-tipped swab (before lubricant use); the vaginal pH of women with VVA is typically greater than 5.0 [4,5]. Examination of the vagina might reveal shortening and narrowing of the vagina, smooth, and thin mucosa along with other vaginal signs (see Table 1) [4,5,11,26,27]. A culture should be obtained if physical examination findings are consistent with infection; a biopsy should be taken for atypical presentation [4]. HCPs uncomfortable with obtaining biopsies should refer to a gynecologist.

MANAGEMENT

Over-the-counter preparations (eg, vaginal lubricants and moisturizers) and prescription therapies have demonstrated effectiveness in managing VVA symptoms [4]. Consistent with principles of shared decision making, treatment and goals should reflect the patient's values and preferences and should be aimed at alleviating bothersome symptoms [4,28,29]. First-line therapies include long-acting vaginal moisturizers and vaginal estrogen for symptoms unrelated to dyspareunia. With symptoms primarily related to sexual activity, stepwise therapy starts with vaginal lubricants and moisturizers. If these measures do not sufficiently alleviate dyspareunia, topical estrogen therapy (TET) is recommended unless contraindicated [4]. Furthermore, although nonhormonal treatments may initially be helpful, VVA is progressive and most likely eventually requires hormonal therapy [14]. Although systemic estrogen is approved by the Food and Drug Administration for symptomatic vaginal atrophy, it is typically insufficient to provide relief of symptoms (especially dyspareunia) requiring concomitant use of TET [18]. If hormone therapy is required solely for symptoms of VVA, topical preparations are recommended [18,30]. Alternative treatments including acupuncture, plant estrogens, soy, chasteberry, ginseng, black cohosh, and the traditional Japanese herbal formula, Kampo, cannot be recommended because they have not been well studied or, when studied, have not demonstrated improvement [4,25]. Women with significant vaginal constriction hindering penetration should be referred to a gynecologist or physical therapy for treatments, such as vaginal dilators and pelvic floor therapy [4].

Nonpharmacologic

Nonhormonal vaginal lubricants and moisturizers provide temporary relief of VVA symptoms but do not have an effect on genital physiologic changes associated with menopause [11]. Women report liking the safety and side effect profile of over-the-counter, nonpharmacologic products for VVA symptoms [12]. Perceived long-term safety benefits, when opting for nonpharmacologic interventions, include concerns about the potential risk for endometrial and breast cancer with hormone therapy [12]. Some evidence exists suggesting that women with a single symptom of VVA or minor bother may experience similar improvement of dryness, dyspareunia, and pruritis with lubricants and moisturizers when compared with TET [2].

Lifestyle modifications

Lifestyle modifications include avoiding vulvar irritants, such as perfumed products, panty liners, menstrual products, and powders, along with vulvar hygiene including wearing loose-fitting cotton underwear and thoroughly drying the genital area after bathing [4,18,25]. Regular sexual activity has also been shown to improve vaginal dryness and maintain vaginal health [4].

Lubricants

Vaginal dryness is one of the most common symptoms in VVA [12,14]. Lubricants are thickening agents (silicone, water, mineral oil, or plant oil based) and are used for quick, short-term relief from vaginal dryness, such as before sexual intercourse [31]. Water-based lubricants, such as Astroglide and K–Y Jelly, are nonstaining and are associated with fewer negative symptoms when compared with silicone-based products [31]. Silicone-based lubricants include Astroglide X and K–Y Intrigue. Lubricants have the potential for irritation and application is messy [14]. Lubricants must be applied routinely to maintain vaginal hydration.

Moisturizers

Vaginal moisturizers hydrate the vaginal mucosa adhering to the vaginal lining and also lower vaginal pH to premenopausal levels [4,31]. Regular use of long-acting moisturizers, ranging from daily to every 2 to 3 days, is included as first-line treatment in women with VVA symptoms related to sexual activity [4,31]. Additional use of lubricants during sexual activity may reduce irritation related to friction [4]. Examples of moisturizers include Replens and Vagisil [4]. As with lubricants, moisturizers have the potential for local irritation and are messy to administer [14].

Patient education

Women should test the moisturizer or lubricant for irritation on a patch of skin for 24 hours before intravaginal application. If dermatitis occurs at the test site, women should be advised to switch to an isomolar product, such as Good Clean, a propylene glycol–free product, such as Good Clean Love, or silicone-based lubricants [4]. Women should also be advised that oil-based products can compromise condom integrity, whereas most water- and silicone-based lubricants are latex safe and appropriate for use with condoms [4].

Pharmacologic

Vaginal estrogen

Nonhormonal treatments can provide relief of symptoms but are likely inadequate for those initially identified with severe symptoms of VVA or as GSM progresses because they do not provide the restorative effects of estrogen [14,18]. When patients present with severe VVA or when nonpharmacologic interventions prove insufficient, TET is widely recognized as the most effective treatment of moderate to severe symptoms with up to 90% of women treated reporting symptom improvement. Women should be given the lowest possible dose that achieves and maintains symptom improvement [4,14,25,32]. Estrogen therapy in postmenopausal women seems to affect primarily estrogen-receptor α in the vagina where estrogen-receptor density is highest [17]. Vaginal estrogen restores epithelial thickness, reestablishes lactobacilli resulting in restoration of an acidic pH, and increases vascularization, which improves vaginal secretions and moisture [32,33]. Additionally, TET is believed to decrease sensory nociceptor neurons in the vagina, which might reduce physical discomfort associated with VVA [17].

Vaginal estrogen is available in cream, gel, tablet, and ring formulations [34]. A 2016 Cochrane Review of randomized trials of menopausal women using intravaginal estrogen preparations found that all of the formulations demonstrated improvement in symptoms over placebo; there is no evidence of a difference in the improvement of symptoms between the various formulations [34]. Maximum benefit of TET is typically obtained within 3 months after initiation of treatment [25].

Adverse effects. Overall, reports of adverse events are low. The most reported adverse events for TET include irritation, burning, pruritis, and vaginal leukorrhea. A small number of women report mastalgia [32].

Safety. A total of 41% of women taking prescription therapies for VVA cite concerns about long-term safety [12]. Endometrial and breast cancer safety are common concerns with exogeneous estrogen administration. The dose of topical required to treat VVA is approximately one-hundredth of the dose of systemic estrogen used for vasomotor symptoms of menopause [18,33]. A transient increase in serum estriol levels following treatment with TET occurs with eventual return to at or lower than the average level for menopausal women [4,32]. Studies demonstrate evidence of an endometrial estrogenic response to TET but no endometrial estrogenic effects at 6- or 12-month follow-up by hysteroscopy and histology [32]. There is no evidence of a difference in an increase in endometrial thickness with tablet compared with creams [34]. Evidence exists that women treated with estrogen creams experience a greater increase in endometrial thickness when compared with a ring. However, higher doses of cream were used in the studies than used in clinical practice [34]. Based on current evidence, concomitant use of progestogen with TET is not recommended [4]. There is insufficient evidence to support annual endometrial surveillance in asymptomatic women using TET; however, studies on endometrial safety have not been established beyond 12 months and any vaginal bleeding requires prompt evaluation [18,25]. Women at high risk for endometrial cancer or using a higher than a typical recommended dose of TET, should be considered for annual transvaginal ultrasound surveillance or progesterone withdrawal [4]. Finally, TET is contraindicated in women with undiagnosed etiology for vaginal or uterine bleeding [4].

A total of 30% of women cite breast cancer risk as a source of concern for use of prescription therapy for VVA [12]. Evidence regarding the safety of TET in women with a history of breast cancer is limited [4]. There is evidence of uterine first-pass effect indicating that intravaginal application results in a preferential effect in the uterus [4]. Additionally, absence of sustained elevated serum estriol levels suggests TET seems to be safe even in women at risk for adverse consequences related to estrogen therapy [32]. It is recommended that women with a history of endometrial or breast cancer who do not respond to nonhormonal treatments for GSM (including VVA) engage in shared decision making with the treating oncologist to explore TET [29,32].

Administration. Initial administration of vaginal estradiol tablets (Vagifem) is one tablet daily for 2 weeks followed by a maintenance dose of one tablet twice weekly. 17β-estradiol cream (Estrace) has a recommended initial dose of 2 to 4 g daily for 1 to 2 weeks followed by a maintenance dose of 1-g dose, one to three times weekly. The 2-mg 17β-estradiol ring (Estring) is inserted intravaginally for 90 days; less frequent administration requirement might improve adherence. Conjugated estrogens (Premarin Vaginal Cream) is dosed 0.5 to 2 g daily for 21 days with a 7-day hiatus for VVA and 0.5 g for 21 days with a maintenance dose of either 7 days off or twice weekly for dyspareunia [4]. No limitations on duration of therapy have been established [4].

Patient education. Education should include information about safety and efficacy of TET. Women should be advised that the estradiol ring may be dislodged with defecation and Valsalva or with intravaginal insertion, such as during intercourse or douching, and that if treatment is discontinued, symptoms are likely to recur [2,4]. Women experiencing any vaginal bleeding should report their symptoms to their HCP immediately.

Estrogen receptor agonist/antagonist
Ospemifene is a novel selective estrogen receptor modulator with unique vaginal effects approved by the Food and Drug Administration for the treatment of moderate to severe menopausal dyspareunia [4,18]. The vaginal effects of ospemifene include improvement in vaginal epithelium and pH, vaginal dryness, and dyspareunia [4,18]. The most frequently reported adverse event are hot flashes [18]. Urinary tract infection, vaginal discharge, vulvar and vaginal yeast infections, nasopharyngitis, and cephalgia are other reported adverse reactions [18].

Safety. Ospemifene (Osphena) has not been found to be associated with venous thrombus embolism (VTE), endometrial hyperplasia, or cancer after 1 year of therapy [4]. However, ospemifene carries the class label precaution for VTE. Ospemifene should not be prescribed for women with a history of breast cancer or women with undiagnosed vaginal bleeding because of lack of long-term studies on endometrial and breast cancer safety [4,29].

Dosing and patient education. Ospemifene is dosed at one 60-mg tablet daily taken with food. Ospemifene should be discontinued for 4 to 6 weeks before surgery associated with VTE risk. Women experiencing any vaginal bleeding should report their symptoms immediately [35].

EVALUATION AND FOLLOW-UP
Improvement of symptoms occurs within a few weeks after initiation of TET and ospemifene; full therapeutic effect is usually achieved by 3 months [4,25]. A follow-up visit at 2 to 4 weeks after initiation is recommended to evaluate treatment adherence, tolerance, and symptom improvement [14]. Lack of response after 12 weeks necessitates exploring other differential diagnoses as described previously [4]. Change in the severity of the baseline most bothersome symptoms initially selected by the woman can be used to evaluate symptom improvement [22]. Change in scores on the VSQ and DIVA questionnaires can also aid in evaluation of treatment efficacy [23,24]. Treatment should be modified if the woman experiences adverse reactions, insufficient improvement, or poor adherence; re-evaluation and monitoring should occur at regular intervals [14]. Women treated with TET who experience any vaginal bleeding must be evaluated for the possibility of endometrial cancer including a transvaginal ultrasound and/or endometrial biopsy [4].

SUMMARY
The genital effects of estrogen depletion on women are highly prevalent and burdensome. A range of effective, safe treatments for VVA are readily available and well within the primary care HCP scope of practice. However, VVA is widely underreported and untreated because of a variety of factors including patient lack of knowledge, communication barriers between women and their HCPs, and clinician discomfort in evaluating and treating VVA. Primary care clinicians, as front-line providers, are well positioned to address this

burdensome condition through education, diagnosis, evaluation, and treatment of VVA, thus improving QOL in the growing population of older adult women.

References

[1] Population aging in the United States a global perspective. Federal Interagency Forum on Aging Related Statistics; 2016. Available at: https://agingstats.gov/images/olderamericans_agingpopulation.pdf. Accessed January 15, 2019.

[2] Rahn DD, Carberry C, Sanses TV, et al. Vaginal estrogen for genitourinary syndrome of menopause: a systematic review. Obstet Gynecol 2014;124(6):1147–56.

[3] Panay N. Genitourinary syndrome of the menopause: dawn of a new era? Climacteric 2015;18(1 supplement):18–22.

[4] The North American Menopause Society. Management of symptomatic vulvovaginal atrophy: 2013 position statement of The North American Menopause Society. Menopause 2013;20(9):888–902.

[5] Phillips NA, Bachmann GA. Genitourinary syndrome of menopause: common problem, effective treatments. Cleve Clin J Med 2018;85(5):390–8.

[6] Wiers SG, Keilman LJ. Improving care for women with urinary incontinence in primary care. J Nurse Pract 2017;13(10):675–80.

[7] Portman DJ, Gass MLS. Genitourinary syndrome of menopause: new terminology for vulvovaginal atrophy from the International Society for the Study of Women's Sexual Health and The North American Menopause Society. Maturitas 2014;79(3):349–54.

[8] Lev-Sagie A. Vulvar and vaginal atrophy: physiology, clinical presentation, and treatment considerations. Clin Obstet Gynecol 2015;58(3):476–91.

[9] Nappi RE, Cucinella L, Martella S, et al. Female sexual dysfunction (FSD): prevalence and impact on quality of life (QoL). Maturitas 2016;94:87–91.

[10] DiBonaventura M, Luo X, Moffatt M, et al. The association between vulvovaginal atrophy symptoms and quality of life among postmenopausal women in the United States and Western Europe. J Womens Health 2015;24(9):713–22.

[11] Kagan R, Rivera E. Restoring vaginal function in postmenopausal women with genitourinary syndrome of menopause. Menopause 2018;25(1):106–8.

[12] Kingsberg SA, Wysocki S, Magnus L, et al. Vulvar and vaginal atrophy in postmenopausal women: findings from the REVIVE (REal women's views of treatment options for menopausal vaginal ChangEs) survey. J Sex Med 2013;10:1790–9.

[13] Nappi RE, Palacios S. Impact of vulvovaginal atrophy on sexual health and quality of life at postmenopause. Climacteric 2014;17(1):3–9.

[14] Kingsberg SA, Krychman ML. Resistance and barriers to local estrogen therapy in women with atrophic vaginitis. J Sex Med 2013;10(6):1567–74.

[15] Krychman M, Graham S, Bernick B, et al. The women's EMPOWER survey: women's knowledge and awareness of treatment options for vulvar and vaginal atrophy remains inadequate. J Sex Med 2017;14(3):425–33.

[16] Baber RJ, Panay N, Fenton AtIWG. 2016 IMS recommendations on women's midlife health and menopause hormone therapy. Climacteric 2016;19(2):109–50.

[17] Derzko C, Elliott S, Lam W. Management of sexual dysfunction in postmenopausal breast cancer patients taking adjuvant aromatase inhibitor therapy. Curr Oncol 2007;14(Suppl 1):S20–40.

[18] Al-Safi ZA, Santoro N. Menopausal hormone therapy and menopausal symptoms. Fertil Steril 2014;101(4):905–15.

[19] Iglesia CB. What's new in the world of postmenopausal sex? Curr Opin Obstet Gynecol 2016;28(5):449–54.

[20] Rhodes KV, Frankel RM, Levinhal N, et al. "You're not a victim of domestic violence, are you?" Provider-patient communication about domestic violence. Ann Intern Med 2007;147:620–7.

[21] McCullers Varner J. Difficult conversations. New Hampshire Nursing News 2012;16.

[22] Weber MA. The effect of vaginal oestriol cream on subjective and objective symptoms of stress urinary incontinence and vaginal atrophy: an international multi-centre pilot study. Gynecol Obstet Invest 2017;82(1):15–21.

[23] Erekson EA, Yip SO, Wedderburn TS, et al. The VSQ: a questionnaire to measure vulvovaginal symptoms in postmenopausal women. Menopause 2013;20(9):978–9.

[24] Huang AJ, Gregorich SE, Kuppermann M, et al. The day-to-day impact of vaginal aging questionnaire: a multidimensional measure of the impact of vaginal symptoms on functioning and well-being in postmenopausal women. Menopause 2015;22(2):144–54.

[25] Calleja-Agiu J, Brincat MP. The urogenital system and the menopause. Climacteric 2015;18(Supplement 1):18–22.

[26] Erekson EA, Fang-Young L, Martin DK, et al. Vulvovaginal symptoms prevalence in postmenopausal women and relationship to other menopausal symptoms and pelvic floor disorders. Menopause 2016;23(4):368–75.

[27] Brotman RM, Shardell MD, Gajer P, et al. Association between the vaginal microbiota, menopause status, and signs of vulvovaginal atrophy. Menopause 2014;21(5):450–8.

[28] Friesen-Storms JHHM, Bours GJJW, van der Weijden T, et al. Shared decision making in chronic care in the context of evidence based practice in nursing. Int J Nurs Stud 2015;52(1):393–402.

[29] Stuenkel C A, Davis S R, Gompel A, et al. Treatment of symptoms of the menopause: an Endocrine Society clinical practice guideline. J Clin Endocrinol Metab 2015;100(11): 3975–4011.

[30] Krychman ML. Vaginal estrogens for the treatment of dyspareunia. J Sex Med 2011;8(3): 666–74.

[31] Edwards D, Panay N. Treating vulvovaginal atrophy/genitourinary syndrome of menopause: how important is vaginal lubricant and moisturizer composition? Climacteric 2016;19(2):151–61.

[32] Rueda C, Osorio AM, Alvellaneda AC, et al. The efficacy and safety of estriol to treat vulvovaginal atrophy in postmenopausal women: a systematic literature review. Climacteric 2017;20(4):321–30.

[33] Pinkerton JV, Kaunitz AM, Manson JE. Vaginal estrogen in the treatment of genitourinary syndrome of menopause and risk of endometrial cancer: an assessment of recent studies provides reassurance. Menopause 2017;24(12):1329–32.

[34] Lethaby A, Ayeleke RO, Roberts H. Local oestrogen for vaginal atrophy in postmenopausal women. Cochrane Database Syst Rev 2016;(8):CD001500.

[35] Epocrates, Inc. Osphena. Available at: https://www.epocrates.com. Accessed January 15, 2019.

[36] MegaLexica. Medical dictionary online. n.d. Available at: https://www.online-medical-dictionary.org/. Accessed September 26, 2018.

[37] Diasio RB. Principles of drug therapy. In: Goldman L, Schaefer AI, editors. Goldman-Cecil medicine. 25th edition. Philadelphia: Saunders; 2016. p. 124–33.e122.

[38] Meczekalski B, Podfigurna-Stopa A, Czyzyk A, et al. Why hypoestrogenism in young women is so important? Archives of Perinatal Medicine 2014;20(2):78–80.

[39] Bowen R. Classification of vaginal epithelial cells. 1998. Available at: http://www.vivo.colostate.edu/hbooks/pathphys/reprod/vc/cells.html. Accessed January 15, 2019.

[40] The Free Medical Dictionary by Farlex. (n.d.). Rugae. Available at: https://medical-dictionary.thefreedictionary.com/rugae. Accessed January 15, 2019.

[41] Medicine.net. (2018). Medical definition of Elastin. Available at: https://www.medicine-net.com/script/main/art.asp?articlekey=24541. Accessed January 15, 2019.

[42] The Free Medical Dictionary by Farlex. (n.d.) Hypeplasia. Available at: https://medical-dictionary.thefreedictionary.com/hyperplasia. Accessed January 15, 2019.

Advances in Family Practice Nursing 1 (2019) 87–97

ADVANCES IN FAMILY PRACTICE NURSING

Approaching Frailty in Primary Care

Deborah Dunn, EdD, MSN, GNP-BC, ACNS-BC, GS C*

The Graduate School, Center for Research, Madonna University, Livonia, MI, USA

Keywords
• Frailty • Assessment • Frailty criteria • Older adults • Physical disability
• Primary care • Frail elderly

Key points

- Frailty is a complex syndrome that affects millions of older adults in the United States.
- Older adults who are frail are 3 to 5 times more susceptible to adverse health events.
- Frailty assessment tools can be easily integrated into the primary care visit.
- Early identification of frailty provides the opportunity to improve patients' physical, functional, and psychosocial well-being and to lengthen the amount of time older adults are able to experience robust health and independent living.

INTRODUCTION

Frailty is a distinct clinical syndrome associated with aging and characterized by decreased strength, endurance, and reduced physiologic reserve and is associated with poor medical outcomes [1]. Frailty can be discretely distinguished from disability and comorbidity, as individuals can be disabled but not frail and may have comorbidities and not be frail [2]. Frailty can and does exist independently from disability and comorbidity. As a clinical syndrome, frailty is classified as a dynamic condition with a hierarchal pattern, with states ranging from "nonfrail" or "robust" to "prefrail," "frail," and "advanced frailty" [3] (Fig. 1).

Studies assessing for the prevalence of frailty among community dwelling older adults have reported that in persons 65 and older, approximately 39%

Disclosure Statement: The author has no commercial or financial conflicts of interest or any funding sources to disclose.

*36600 Schoolcraft Road, Livonia, MI 48150-1176. E-mail address: ddunn@madonna.edu

https://doi.org/10.1016/j.yfpn.2018.12.003
2589-420X/19/© 2019 Elsevier Inc. All rights reserved.

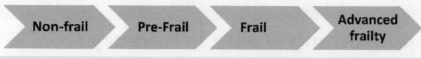

Fig. 1. States of frailty.

were robust, 45% were prefrail, and 15% were frail [3]. The highest rates of frailty prevalence were seen among those living in residential care, persons of lower income, women, racial and ethnic minorities, and adults over the age of 80 [3]. According to the US Census Bureau, the population of persons 65 and older will double over the next 3 decades, and those aged 80 and older are expected to triple [4]. As the US population of older adults escalates, there is a growing need for frailty screening and intervention in order to improve care for this most vulnerable segment of older adults.

FRAILTY ASSESSMENT
Frailty assessment of older adults in primary care provides an opportunity for frailty identification and stratification. Once frailty is identified, nurse practitioners (NPs) can construct a plan of care with interventions aimed at preventing frailty or effectively reducing the degree of frailty in order to reduce adverse health outcomes, morbidity, and mortality and extend the span of robust health [1]. Growing evidence has supported the usefulness of frailty assessment tools in identifying levels of frailty and predicting future or worsening outcomes, such as activities of daily living (ADL), dependency, health decline, adverse outcomes following outpatient emergency visits, increased hospitalization, prolonged length of stay, postoperative complications, nosocomial complications, likelihood of discharge to a care facility, and increased mortality [5–8].

The Frailty Phenotype (FP) is a widely accepted and applied definition of frailty [1]. The FP recognizes frailty as a syndrome and has 5 assessment criteria for the presence of frailty; these include weight loss, exhaustion, low activity, slow walking speed, and weak hand grip [1,5]. The Cardiovascular Health Study Frailty Screening Scale (CHSFSS) is a validated assessment tool that uses these 5 criteria; scores range from 0 (best) to 5 (worst) with one point scored for each criteria present and rate persons as "prefrail" if they have 1 or 2 criteria present and "frail" if 3 or more of the criteria are present (Table 1). The "FRAIL" questionnaire is another quick and easy-to-use frailty assessment tool with 5 rating criteria: fatigue, resistance, aerobic capacity, illnesses, and weight loss [1,6]. FRAIL questionnaire scores range from 0 (best) to 5 (worst), with a one-point rating for each criteria present; a score of 3 to 5 indicates "frailty," 1 to 2 "prefrail," and 0 "robust" [6] (Table 2).

The Clinical Frailty Scale (CFS) is a convenient third option for clinical use. The CFS is a validated tool that bases frailty assessment on clinical judgment with 9 descriptive categories; 1 (very fit) to 9 (terminally ill) and contains

Table 1
Cardiovascular health study frailty screening scale

1	Weight loss	Unintentional weight loss of ≥ 10 pounds in past year or $\leq 10\%$ of weight at age 60
2	Exhaustion	Self-report of fatigue or unusual tiredness in the past month
3	Low activity	Frequency and duration of physical activities (walking, doing strenuous household chores, doing strenuous outdoor chores, dancing, bowling, exercise)
4	Slowness	Walking 4 m ≥ 7 s if height ≤ 159 cm or ≥ 6 s if height ≥ 159 cm[a]
5	Weakness	Grip strength (kg) for body mass index (kg/m^2)

Prefrail, 1 or 2; frail, ≥ 3.
[a]Data for older women (lowest 20th percentile).
Adapted from Morley JE, Vellas B, Van Kan AG, et al. Frailty consensus: a call to action. J Am Med Dir Assoc 2013;14 (6):394; with permission.

accompanying figures for clinician reference [8]. In the Canadian Study of Health and Aging, the CFS demonstrated good construct and criterion validity in a 5-year prediction of adverse health events, institutionalization, and death [9]. Further research using the CFS identified score ranges for the clinical descriptors with a score of 1 to 4 "nonfrail," 5 to 6 "mild to moderately frail," and 7 to 8 "severely frail"; these categories correlated with longer hospital length of stay [10]. Primary care assessment of frailty positively aids clinicians in identifying older adult patients at risk for hospital complications and provides an opportunity for preemptive health protective care planning.

CASE REVIEW
The 4 cases discussed illustrate how frailty assessment aids in identifying older adults at risk for adverse health events and can provide guidance for protective health care planning and intervention across care settings.

Case 1
An 84-year-old woman with a history of asthma, osteoporosis, osteoarthritis (OA), severe kyphosis, and hypertension (HTN) is recovering in a short-stay

Table 2
FRAIL questionnaire

1	Fatigue	Are you fatigued? "All of the time" or "most of the time"
2	Resistance	Difficulty walking up one flight of steps alone without resting or aids
3	Aerobic	Walk 1 block alone without aids or resting
4	Illnesses	5 or more illnesses
5	Loss of weight	Weight loss of $\geq 5\%$ in the past 12 mo

Robust: 0; prefrail: 1 to 2; frail: 3 to 5.
Adapted from Morley JE, Malmstrom TK, Miller DK. A simple frailty questionnaire (FRAIL) predicts outcomes in middle aged African Americans. J Nutr Health Aging 2012;16(7):601–8; with permission.

rehabilitation center following hospitalization for a fall, intractable back pain, vertebral compression fracture, and recent kyphoplasty. There is no weight loss. She denies unusual fatigue. She lives with her son, who works during the day. She is able to self-medicate, is independent in ADL, receives assistance with instrumental activities of daily living (IADLs), is ambulatory, and is able to walk independently (>600 feet).

Case 2

A 75-year-old man with a history of HTN, tobacco smoking, dyslipidemia, OA of both knees, and surgical history of a left total knee arthroplasty is hospitalized for acute syncope, aortic aneurysm dissection, and surgical repair. He is a widower, lives alone, and has 2 adult children who are married and live in another state. Before hospitalization, he was driving, independent in IADLs and ADLs. He was active and worked out at the senior center with friends 3 days a week. Postoperatively, he reports significant fatigue, low appetite, and fear of falling when walking to the bathroom.

Case 3

An 80-year-old woman with a history of HTN, diverticulitis, lumbar spine OA, and bilateral cataract surgery is seen in the clinic for a 3-month primary care visit. Her weight has decreased 10% in the past year, and she reports this as unintentional weight loss. She walks 1 mile daily and lives with her husband in a senior independent living apartment. She describes herself as active and enjoys volunteering at the local elementary school and coaching reading once a month in third-grade classrooms.

Case 4

Case 4 is an 82-year-old man who is a resident of an assisted living facility. Past medical history includes insulin-dependent diabetes type 2, HTN, chronic atrial fibrillation, chronic obstructive pulmonary disease, dyslipidemia, chronic renal failure, macular degeneration, ischemic stroke with residual left-hand weakness, and gait/balance disorder. He walks short distances with a walker, cannot climb stairs, needs assistance with medication setup, does not drive, is able to perform ADLs but requires rest periods following hygiene and toileting activities. Serial weights show he has experienced a 5% weight loss in the past 6 months.

In the case examples provided, cases 1 and 3 present older adults with a "prefrail" state. These older adults are likely to benefit from referral to a Geriatrician or Gerontological Specialist for comprehensive geriatric assessment (CGA) and management. In addition to using the information provided through frailty assessment, the specialist along with the interdisciplinary team can perform targeted assessments to identify specific areas to maximize functional status and promote wellness. Examples include optimizing home safety, medication management, nutritional status, physical activity, and social well-being.

Case 3 demonstrates a 75-year-old man with frailty who would benefit from care in an Acute Care for the Elderly (ACE) hospital unit. ACE units provide specialized supportive care to hospitalized older adults as they recover from acute health conditions and care interventions that reduce functional decline and support safe discharge to home or an appropriate environment while reducing chances of readmission to the hospital [11]. In case 4, this 82-year-old man demonstrates frailty, because he has greater than 5 active illnesses, functional impairment, weight loss, and fatigue. Goals of care should focus on reducing vulnerability to health decline, injury, social isolation, and repeat hospitalizations. Coordinated primary care and geriatric specialist care can provide a comprehensive management plan to reduce functional decline and preserve independence. The Program of All-Inclusive Care for the Elderly (PACE) is another care option to consider. PACE is a community-based program that provides comprehensive coordinated care by an interdisciplinary team aimed at supporting vulnerable older adults in their efforts to remain in their preferred care setting, thus avoiding long-term care placement [11,12].

THE PRIMARY CARE CLINICAL VISIT

A proposed approach to the primary care clinical visit for frailty assessment is to (1) establish who should be targeted for frailty screening, (2) select a screening tool, (3) use criteria-based diagnosis (ie, robust/nonfrail; prefrail; frail; advanced frailty), and (4) establish goals and determine the management plan through patient-centered decision making [1].

Who should you screen?

Any older adult aged 70 or older should be screened annually; those with unintentional weight loss of 5% or greater screen on a regular basis, and any older adult patient planning an elective surgery [2,8–10].

Which screening tool should you use?

Choose a screening tool suitable to your clinical practice. The CHSFSS, the FRAIL questionnaire, and the CFS are 3 well-validated tools to choose from that are useful for rapid frailty screening across care settings [1,5,6,8,9]. In addition, the American Geriatric Society Geriatrics Evaluation and Management Tools provide a comprehensive yet succinct guideline that outlines frailty screening, provides a screening tool, establishes a history and physical examination guide, suggests laboratory tests to consider, and provides a management guide of interventions for prevention to treatment of frailty [13].

How do you diagnose frailty?

The screening instrument the NP uses will determine the frailty classification you should assign: robust/nonfrail; prefrail; or frail. Furthermore, the screening tool classification will help to determine the direction of management and focused interventions to target deficits associated with frailty.

How should you approach care management?

A positive screen for frailty should prompt thorough assessment, with the gold standard being comprehensive geriatric evaluation and management (GEM) [1,13,14]. CGA provides a multidimensional assessment that incorporates a multidisciplinary team approach and provides a wide range of medical, functional, psychological, social, and quality-of-life (QOL) assessment data [1,15]. This broad approach is able to identify possible modifiable, reversible, and/ or precipitating factors of frailty that can be targeted for intervention and management. In addition, CGA provides essential clinical data related to the 5 frailty assessment areas (ie, CHSFSS: weight loss; fatigue; activity; slowness; weakness; or FRAIL: fatigue; resistance; aerobic; illnesses; weight loss) [1,5,6].

FRAILTY TREATMENT AND MANAGEMENT

Treatment goals should be mutually established between the clinician, the patient, and the patient's caregivers. The overall goal of frailty treatment and management is to improve physical, functional, and psychosocial well-being and to lengthen the amount of time older adults are able to experience robust health and independent living. Some specific goals for frailty prevention and amelioration to discuss with your patients include the following:

- Maintaining or restoring physical strength, exercise tolerance, and mobility
- Maintaining or restoring nutritional status and healthy weight
- Reducing polypharmacy
- Maintaining or restoring environmental safety
- Avoiding falls and injury
- Maintaining or restoring level of ADL function
- Maintaining capacity for independent or preferred living environment
- Decreasing vulnerability to stress
- Avoiding depression and social isolation
- Avoiding excess morbidity

EVIDENCED-BASED TREATMENT APPROACHES

Prospective cohort studies have shown frailty to be a progressive syndrome with transitions from lesser degrees of frailty to greater degrees of frailty and with functional decline being common [16–18]. Because frailty is a progressive syndrome, management must be targeted, sustained, and ongoing throughout the trajectory of frailty [11,14,16,19]. Interventions and their effectiveness at interrupting frailty progression and restoring older adults to a nonfrail or lesser state of frailty have been studied.

Interventions showing the most positive effects on frailty to date are (1) physical activity/exercise [17–22], (2) nutritional support to prevent weight loss, (3) coordinated care provided by an interdisciplinary team [19,23], (4) supportive community based programs such as PACE [19,24] for frail community dwelling older adults, and (5) when hospitalization is required, elder-sensitive care provided on an ACE unit reduces adverse health events [19,25,26].

MANAGING PREFRAILTY

Although there is a paucity of literature regarding evidence-based interventions for the prevention of frailty, expert opinion suggests implementing some of the same treatments suggested for frailty management. These treatments include (1) regular exercise (aerobic and resistance), at least 45 to 60 minutes of aerobic activity 3 times a week along with resistance training 2 times a week [1,16,27–29]; (2) lifestyle modification (ie, smoking cessation) [11]; (3) treatment of known chronic illnesses [11,16]; (4) health screenings [1,11,28]; (5) preventive health maintenance [1,27]; (6) minimizing polypharmacy [13,30]; and (7) nutrition supplementation [1,2,11,13,14,16]. Prefrailty interventions should be continued across the spectrum of frailty and assessed for their benefit and/or burden if frailty progresses [11]. Fig. 2 provides a summary of care interventions across the spectrum of frailty.

MANAGING MODERATE FRAILTY

Older persons demonstrating moderate frailty have been shown to benefit from structured physical activity programs. In a study of 188 community-dwelling moderately frail older adults participating in an in-home physical therapy program, Gill and colleagues [17] found significant reduction in physical impairment, frailty, and functional status decline in the treatment group. Similarly, in a study of 610 community-dwelling frail older adults participating in a community-based exercise program, Yamada and colleagues [30] found older adults experienced a reduction in frailty progression and improved physical function. A systematic review by Theou and colleagues [31] found that structured exercise programs (60 minutes 3 times per week) lasting ≥5 months were beneficial for frail older adults and slowed the overall progression of frailty (see Fig. 2).

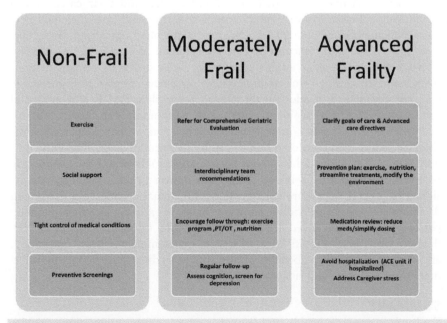

Fig. 2. Frailty interventions by stage.

Because frailty is a multisystem syndrome, a combination of interventions is needed to fully affect frailty progression. Exercise plus nutritional interventions shows promise in ameliorating frailty [32,33]. Nutritional supplementation that includes adequate amounts of calories, proteins (1.0–1.5 g/kg/d), and micronutrients has been shown to increase weight, muscle mass, handgrip strength, and improve overall muscle function in frail elders [33,34].

Coordinated care delivered by NPs with geriatric expertise, coupled with interdisciplinary team management, is essential for optimal care of moderately frail older adults. Interdisciplinary care models have shown success in addressing the multidimensional and complex health concerns of vulnerable frail older adults. Through CGA, and GEM models of care, frailty and other geriatric syndromes are readily recognized and addressed along with on-going primary care comanagement of chronic health conditions, and continued supportive and preventative health care interventions.

MANAGING ADVANCED FRAILTY

As frailty progresses, the older adult is at greater risk for health deterioration, so the benefits and burdens of frailty care interventions must be weighed carefully. In many cases, these interventions will continue to be beneficial. Focusing care on health protection, reducing risk for falls, avoiding polypharmacy, supporting nutrition, and encouraging an exercise plan that is gauged to the older adult's level of tolerance will help to stabilize frailty and reduce its progression.

Goals of care should be reviewed annually and regularly with any change in health status. Active engagement of the older adult and their caregivers in monitoring adherence to care interventions and revisiting care goals will help guide patient-centered optimal care. Because of the often complex and multiple conditions older adults encounter, care coordination should be a top priority. Clarifying the frail older adult's care preferences, desire to remain in their own home for care, as well as preferences regarding hospital and end-of-life care are essential to developing the management plan. PACE is a successful model of care that is available to older adults with multiple chronic conditions or those who are nursing home eligible but desiring to receive comparable long-term care services in their own home [24]. In the event of acute illness and hospitalization, frail older adults have been shown to benefit from acute care received on hospital ACE units. These units deliver geriatric-friendly care designed to prevent acute-care complications, functional decline, and worsening disability as well as providing comprehensive proactive discharge planning [26,27]. Last, in advanced frailty, advanced-care directives should be addressed, and there should be a focus on maintaining comfort, autonomy, and dignity. Burdens and benefits of care should be discussed, along with information on palliative and hospice care options.

SUMMARY

Frailty is a growing health problem of concern; as the population of older adults expands, NPs will undoubtedly encounter an increasing number of frail elderly patients in their practices. Frailty is a largely age-related progressive condition once thought to be untreatable but now known to be amenable to improvement with focused treatment strategies. Valid and user-friendly assessment tools are now available for accurate frailty screening. Early recognition of older adults at risk for frailty or in a frail state provides an opportunity for NPs to intervene and interrupt the progression of frailty.

Several interventions are available for the prevention and/or treatment of frailty. Because of the multidimensional nature of frailty, NPs must apply multiple interventions in order to prevent frailty in at-risk older adults, or to transition the older adult with frailty from a frail state to a nonfrail or less frail state and thereby reduce vulnerability. Physical activity, nutritional supplementation, health protection, and chronic illness management interventions play an important role in preventing and treating frailty. Comprehensive geriatric models of care, such as CGA and GEM, are particularly helpful in the care of frail older adults. These models of care provide access to the multidisciplinary health care team, and such care has been shown to foster improvement in health status, to reduce mortality, disability, and negative health outcomes, as well as to increase care adherence, satisfaction with care, and QOL.

IMPLICATIONS FOR PRACTICE

This article demonstrates that primary care NPs have a major role to play in the identification and treatment of frailty. Screening for frailty is an essential component in the care of older adults. NPs can contribute to fostering robust health in their older adult practice population and to ameliorating frailty through a variety of practice strategies. Some suggestions include the following:

- Provide frailty prevention and treatment educational materials (American Geriatrics Society handout) in the waiting room and clinic rooms to raise patient and caregiver awareness about the negative health effects of frailty and need for screening and treatment.
- Encourage engagement in community activities that promote senior health, such as exercise groups at local recreation or senior centers, churches, and hospital's community outreach programs.
- Develop a systematic process for frailty assessment, diagnosis, intervention, and referral.
- Consider adding frailty assessment to the electronic health record, with added pop-up alerts for patients who meet criteria when frailty assessment would be appropriate.
- Perform frailty screening on all older adults aged ≥70 annually, on older adults who have a health status change, and on those undergoing elective surgery.
- Consult geriatric services in your area, develop a relationship with CGA and GEM providers. Refer patients to these services as needed.
- Evaluate patients with functional limitations and/or multiple chronic conditions for appropriateness of care in a PACE program.
- When hospitalization occurs, consider older adults, especially those with frailty, for acute care admission to an ACE unit. Advocate for hospitals in your service area to institute an ACE unit if they do not have one.

- Nurture your rehabilitation medicine, home care, palliative, and hospice care provider relationships to better enable easy referral and a sense of familiarity that you can convey to your patients and their caregivers.

Adding these care strategies to the care of older adults in your practice will better enable you to meet the multidimensional care needs of older adults, especially those with frailty.

References

[1] Morley JE, Vellas B, Van Kan AG, et al. Frailty consensus: a call to action. J Am Med Dir Assoc 2013;14(6):392–7.

[2] Fried LP, Ferrucci L, Darer J, et al. Untangling the concepts of disability, frailty, and comorbidity: implications for improved targeting and care. J Gerontol 2004;59(3):255–63.

[3] Bandeen-Roche K, Seplaki CL, Huang J, et al. Frailty in older adults: a nationally representative profile in the United States. J Gerontol A Biol Sci Med Sci 2015;70(11):1427–34.

[4] He W, Goodkind D, Kowal P, U.S. Census Bureau. International population reports, P95/16-1, an aging world: 2015. Washington (DC): U.S. Government Publishing Office; 2016.

[5] Fried L, Tangen CM, Walston J, et al. Frailty in older adults: evidence for a phenotype. J Gerontol 2001;56(3):146–56.

[6] Morley JE, Malmstrom TK, Miller DK. A simple frailty questionnaire (FRAIL) predicts outcomes in middle aged African americans. J Nutr Health Aging 2012;16(7):601–8.

[7] Hastings NS, Purser JP, Johnson KS, et al. Frailty predicts some but not all adverse outcomes in older adults discharged from the emergency department. J Am Geriatr Soc 2008;56:1651–7.

[8] Makary MA, Segev DL, Pronovost PJ, et al. Frailty as a predictor of surgical outcomes in older patients. J Am Coll Surg 2010;210(6):901–8.

[9] Rockwood K, Song X, MacKnight C, et al. A global clinical measure of fitness and frailty in elderly people. CMAJ 2005;173(5):489–95.

[10] Juma S, Taabazuing MM, Montero-Odasso M. Clinical frailty scale in an acute medicine unit: a simple tool that predicts length of stay. Can Geriatr J 2016;19(2):34–9.

[11] Espinoza S, Walston JD. Frailty in older adults: insights and interventions. Cleve Clin J Med 2005;72(12):1105–12.

[12] Gonzalez L. A focus on the program of all-inclusive care for the elderly (PACE). J Aging Soc Policy 2017; https://doi.org/10.1080/08959420.2017.1281092.

[13] American Geriatrics Society. Frailty: geriatrics evaluation & management tools 2012. Available at: www.americangeriatrics.org. Accessed July 28, 2018.

[14] Fairhall N, Langron C, Sherrington C, et al. Treating frailty-a practical guide. BMC Med 2011;9(83); https://doi.org/10.1186/1741-7015-9-83.

[15] Elsawy B, Higgins KE. The geriatric assessment. Am Fam Physician 2011;83(1):48–56.

[16] Mitnitski A, Song X, Skoog I, et al. Relative fitness and frailty of elderly men and women in developed countries and their relationship with mortality. J Am Geriatr Soc 2005;53:2184–9.

[17] Gill TM, Baker DI, Gottschalk M, et al. A program to prevent functional decline in physically frail, elderly persons who live at home. N Engl J Med 2002;347(14):1068–74.

[18] Gill TM, Gahbauer EA, Allore HG, et al. Transitions between frailty states among community-living older persons. Arch Intern Med 2006;166:418–23.

[19] Xue Qian-Li. The frailty syndrome: definition and natural history. Clin Geriatr Med 2011;27:1–15.

[20] Hubbard RE, Fallah N, Searle SD, et al. Impact of exercise in community-dwelling older adults. PLoS One 2009;4(7):e6174.

[21] Cesari M, Vellas B, Hsu Fang-Chi, et al. A physical activity intervention to treat the frailty syndrome in older persons – results from the LIFE-P study. J Gerontol A Biol Sci Med Sci 2015;70(2):216–22.

[22] McIssac DI, Jen T, Mookerji N, et al. Interventions to improve the outcomes of frail people having surgery: a systematic review. PLoS One 2017;12(12):e0190071.

[23] Ellis G, Gradner M, Tsiachristas A, et al. Comprehensive geriatric assessment for older adults admitted to hospital. Cochrane Database Syst Rev 2017;(9):CD006211.

[24] Beauchamp J, Cheh V, Schmitz , et al. The effect of the program of all-inclusive care for the elderly (PACE) on quality 2008 Avaliable at: https://www.cms.gov/Research-Statistics-Data-and-Systems/Statistics-Trends-and Reports/Reports/downloads/beauchamp_2008.pdf. Accessed August 28, 2018.

[25] Counsell SR, Holder CM, Liebenauer LL, et al. Effects of multicomponent intervention on functional outcomes and process of care in hospitalized older patients: a randomized controlled trial of acute care for elders (ACE) in a community hospital. J Am Geriatr Soc 2000;48(12): 1572–81.

[26] Flood KL, Booth K, Pierlussi E, et al. Acute care for elders. In: Malone ML, Capezuti E, Palmer R, editors. Geriatrics models of care: bringing "best practice" to an aging America. New York: Springer; 2015. p. 3–23.

[27] Ko FC. The clinical care of frail, older adults. Clin Geriatr Med 2011;27:89–100.

[28] Lally F, Crome P. Understanding frailty. Postgrad Med J 2007;83:16–20.

[29] Uchmanowicz I, Jankowska-Polanska B, Wleklik M, et al. Frailty syndrome: nursing interventions. SAGE Open Nurs 2018;4:1–11.

[30] Yamada M, Arai H, Sonoda T, et al. Community-based exercise program is cost-effective by preventing care and disability in Japanese frail older adult. J Am Med Dir Assoc 2012;13: 507–11.

[31] Theou O, Stathokostas L, Roland K, et al. The effectiveness of exercise interventions for the management of frailty: a systematic review. J Aging Res 2011; https://doi.org/10.4061/2011/569194.

[32] Paddon-Jones D. Perspective: exercise and protein supplementation in frail elders. J Am Med Dir Assoc 2013;14:73–4.

[33] Tieland M, Dirks, Van der Zwaluw N, et al. Protein supplementation increases muscle mass gain during prolonged resistance-type exercise training in frail elderly people: a randomized, double-blind, placebo-controlled trial. J Am Med Dir Assoc 2012;13:713–9.

[34] Morley ME, Argiles JM, Evans WJ, et al. Nutritional recommendations for the management of sarcopenia. J Am Med Dir Assoc 2010;11:391–6.

Advances in Family Practice Nursing 1 (2019) 99–115

ADVANCES IN FAMILY PRACTICE NURSING

ELSEVIER
MOSBY

Recognizing and Addressing Elder Abuse in the Primary Care Setting

Natalie R. Baker, DNP, ANP-BC, GNP-BC, GS-C[a],*,
Jennifer Kim, DNP, GNP-BC, GS-C, FNAP[b]

[a]University of Alabama at Birmingham School of Nursing, 1720 Second Avenue South, Birmingham, AL, USA; [b]Vanderbilt University School of Nursing, 461 21st Avenue South, Nashville, TN, USA

Keywords

• Elder mistreatment • Elder abuse • Neglect • Financial exploitation

Key points

• Elder abuse varies in its type, frequency, and intensity and is most often perpetrated by an adult child, spouse, or partner.
• There are both provider and patient barriers that contribute to the problem of underreporting of elder abuse.
• Elder abuse risk factors fall into 4 domains: victim, perpetrator, relationship, and environmental.
• The Elder Abuse Suspicion Index, Hwalke-Sengstock Elder Abuse Screening Test, Vulnerability to Abuse Screening Scale, and Elder Abuse Inventory are all screening tools with established validity in primary care.

A ging is associated with a disruption in health that further results in older adults' increased use of health care resources. This translates to an increased likelihood of interacting with a nurse practitioner (NP) in various outpatient settings. In 2016, it was estimated that 46.2 million Americans were age 65 or older and that 35.7% of this age group had at least 1 disability [1]. Ortman and associates [2] project that 83.7 million older adults will be living in the United States by 2050. The World Health Organization

The authors do not have any financial relationships to disclose.

*Corresponding author. E-mail address: nrbaker@uab.edu

https://doi.org/10.1016/j.yfpn.2018.12.004

estimates that 1 in 6 older adults have been abused in the past year; however, only approximately 4% of elder abuse is reported [3]. During patient encounters, NPs should be vigilant for signs/symptoms that suggest the possibility of elder abuse.

Elder abuse, as defined by World Health Organization, is "a single, or repeated act, or lack of appropriate action, occurring within any relationship where there is an expectation of trust which causes harm or distress to an older person" (para 1) [3]. There are different forms of abuse, some without visual signs (Table 1) [4]. A random sampling of 5777 adults age 60 and older residing in the continental United States revealed that 11.4% of respondents (n = 589) had experienced at least 1 episode of abuse during the previous year [5]. A 2017 systematic review and metaanalysis of published prevalence studies within the community revealed that the overall global prevalence of elder abuse was 15.7%: physical 6%, sexual 0.9%, psychological 11.6%, financial 6.8%, and neglect 4.2% [6].

Table 1
Types of elder abuse and neglect

Type	Definition	Examples
Physical	Use of physical force that results in illness, injury, pain, functional impairment, emotional distress, or death	Hitting, pushing, stomping, scratching, biting, shaking, kicking, choking, burning
Sexual	Any type of unwanted or forced sexual interaction, regardless if genitalia is touched; any sexual act when a person has diminished capacity and is unable to give consent	Attempted or completed penile penetration of vulva or anus; hand, finger, or object penetration of anus or genital opening; mouth contact with penis, vulva, or anus; intentional unwanted touching of genitalia, anus, groin, breasts, inner thighs, or buttocks
Psychological	Verbal or nonverbal behavior that causes mental anguish or pain, or emotional fear or distress	Insulting, name calling, threatening to place in nursing home, isolation from friends and family
Financial	Unauthorized or improper use of an older adult's resources for the benefit of someone other than the older adult	Forgery, misuse or theft of money or possessions; coercion to relinquish money or possessions; improper use of guardianship or power of attorney
Neglect	Failure to protect an older adult from harm, or the failure to meet needs for essential medical care, nutrition, hydration, and basic activities of daily living or shelter that results in a serious risk of compromised health and safety	Not providing adequate nutrition, hygiene, clothing, shelter, or necessary health care; not preventing exposure to unsafe activities and environments

From Centers for Disease Control and Prevention. Elder abuse: definitions. Available at: https://www.cdc.gov/violenceprevention/elderabuse/definitions.html. Accessed August 30, 2018.

RISK FACTORS

Although no older adult is immune from potential abuse, individuals with cognitive, physical, or psychological impairments are at increased risk [5,7]. Notably, studies have shown that minorities and individuals with dementia are especially vulnerable to abuse [7]. Multifactorial etiologies contribute to increased elder abuse risk and can be categorized into 4 domains: victim, perpetrator, relationship, and environmental [8]. Family members account for 90% of all reported elder abuse cases occurring in the home; adult children, spouses and partners are the most likely family offenders (Box 1) [3].

MANDATORY REPORTING

Victims rarely report elder abuse to law enforcement agencies or health care providers for reasons such as fear of retaliation, embarrassment, protection

---

Box 1: Risk factors for elder abuse and neglect

Victim

- Cognitive impairment (ie, dementia, intellectual disability)
- Behavioral issues (ie, loud outbursts, psychiatric illness)
- Functional dependency (ie, feeding assistance, unsteady gait)
- Frailty (ie, frequent acute illnesses)
- Income (ie, poverty, wealthy)
- Minority ethnicity
- Social isolation or loneliness
- Incontinence
- Alcohol use
- Lack of regular primary care provider

Perpetrator (caregiver)

- Caregiver burden or stress
- Inexperience
- Reluctance to assume caregiver role
- Substance abuse or gambling problem
- Financial difficulties
- Behavioral or psychiatric illness
- Cognitive impairment

Relationship

- Family disharmony
- Conflictual relationships

Environmental

- Lack of social support

From Johannesen M, LoGuidice D. Elder abuse: a systematic review of risk factors in community-dwelling elders. Age Ageing 2013;42:292–8.

of the abuser, or mental incompetence [3]. With few exceptions, NPs practicing within the United States are mandatory reporters of suspected abuse [9]. The Stetson University College of Law (https://www.stetson.edu/law/academics/elder/ecpp/statutory-updates.php) maintains updated statutory information on all US state and territory adult protection statutes, including a list of mandatory reporters and agencies to be contacted. Mandatory reporters are not required to prove elder abuse, but must report signs/symptoms of such episodes and make timely notification to appropriate agencies.

ELDER ABUSE EXAMPLES: CASE STUDIES
Neglect and financial exploitation
Annie King is a frail, 80-year-old widow. She does not drive, uses a walker with ambulation, and needs assistance with housecleaning and meal preparation. She met Jessica at church several months ago. Jessica has been living with Annie while she looks for employment. In lieu of paying rent, Jessica provides care for Annie, including running errands and driving her to church and appointments. Annie gave her access to her bank card and password, because Jessica said it would make purchasing groceries, toiletries, and her prescription medications much easier. Unbeknownst to Annie, Jessica has been taking large amounts of cash from her bank account to pay for her own personal expenses.

Annie recently had a bad fall at home, sustaining a thoracic vertebral fracture. The health care provider in the emergency department prescribed hydrocodone and told her to follow-up with her PCP. Not wanting to take an opioid, she never filled her prescription; when she presented to her PCP, she was in severe pain. The NP checked the Controlled Substance Monitoring Database, which indicated a prescription for hydrocodone had been filled 3 days prior. A follow-up call to the pharmacy revealed that Jessica picked up the hydrocodone but told the pharmacist she did not have money to pick up Annie's other prescriptions (metoprolol, lisinopril, atorvastatin), which had not been filled in 6 weeks.

Annie tells her NP that she fell in the hallway of her home while trying to transport the bucket from a portable commode to the bathroom. Jessica sets the commode up in the living room for her because she is often not at home to help her to the bathroom; she is ostensibly looking for employment or running errands. Annie's blood pressure is elevated (180/92 mm Hg) and she has lost 8 pounds since her visit 2 months ago. She is disheveled, has poor hygiene, and is disengaged, but denies depression. Annie adamantly denies that Jessica is harming her, reporting that she is "trying her best." Jessica is not at the NP visit. Annie used a medical ride share van for transportation to today's visit.

Physical
Harold Jones is an 83-year-old nursing home resident with frontotemporal lobe dementia. He often has unpredictable behaviors and aggressive outbursts, which are more pronounced at night. He has recently lost weight. His family

comes to the facility at mealtime to encourage oral intake, but when they are not there, he often refuses to eat. Several certified nursing assistants force feed him out of frustration by his "childish behavior" and out of fear that the family might blame them for any further weight loss. At night, Harold often tries to get out of bed unassisted. His bed alarm alerts staff at least a dozen times every evening. When the nursing home is short staffed, the certified nursing assistants and nurses apply soft wrist restraints, so they do not have to keep coming into his room to turn the bed alarm off. Their behavior does not comply with restraint use requirements; Harold's family does not know he is being restrained. The restraints cause Harold much distress. He often thrashes about in bed, trying to get out of them. He has developed bruising and abrasions around both wrists. He has also developed excoriations and bruising on both arms from his repeated movements with the restraints in place.

Sexual

Edith Brown is a 68-year-old woman with intellectual disabilities and mental health issues. She lived with her mother who managed all aspects of her care until her mother's death 1 year ago. At the time of her mother's death, Edith moved in with her younger cousin Marty and Marty's 2 adult children, Linda and Frank. Marty leaves Edith in the care of her children when she is at work during the day. Linda and Frank both work part time, and Linda's boyfriend often stays with Edith when no one else is available. After several months, Marty noticed a change in Edith; she had become more withdrawn and started resisting help with bathing and dressing. Marty noted a foul-smelling vaginal discharge, which prompted a visit to the NP's office for evaluation.

The NP notes that Edith is very guarded during the physical examination and flinches when touched in the suprapubic region. A gynecologic examination is done, including testing for sexually transmitted infections. The rapid chlamydia test is positive. The NP immediately calls the clinic director and the authorities. Edith does not return to her cousin's home. After a full investigation, it is discovered that Linda's boyfriend had been having nonconsensual sexual intercourse with Edith.

Psychological

Frank and Estelle Washington are a retired couple in their 70s who live in a middle-class neighborhood. A year ago, Estelle developed a rare autoimmune condition that has left her debilitated. Her PCP and specialists have not been able to find an effective treatment and have encouraged her to seek care at the regional academic medical center. The Washingtons have spent much of their savings paying her medical bills and have little money left. Frank is frustrated, and often yells at his wife, blaming her for causing their financial stresses. He has told her that he does not think anything is truly wrong with her, and he often threatens that he will divorce her if she does not improve. He also threatens to return to the work force, stating "You'll have to take care of yourself." When she had a urinary incontinence episode, he yelled at her, calling her a "baby" telling her, "Now I have to spend more money on diapers for you." A neighbor came over later in the day, at which time Frank brought the subject up, calling his wife "pathetic." Estelle cries about this much of the time, which further fuels her husband's abusive behavior.

SCREENING AND ASSESSMENT
Screening
There are differing expert opinions concerning the frequency with which screening should be conducted, because their effectiveness is debated, and there are both potential benefits and harms associated with screening [10]. Screening is important, because it leads to a more in-depth assessment when the NP notes signs/symptoms of potential abuse. Although there are approximately 17 published elder abuse screening tools that may be used in different clinical settings, there is no gold standard, because more research needs to be conducted to rigorously evaluate and validate all tools (Box 2).

In 2013, the Centers for Medicare and Medicaid Services hosted the Elder Mistreatment Symposium at which time 3 elder abuse screening tools were identified and encouraged for use: the Elder Abuse Suspicion Index, the Hwalek-Sengstock Elder Abuse Screening Test, and the Vulnerability to Abuse Screening Scale. These tools were acknowledged for their ability to assess for more than 1 type of abuse, for the measures' specifications, and for the focus

Box 2: Potential benefits and harms of screening for elder abuse

Potential benefits	Potential harms
It is essential for the early detection, treatment, and prevention of elder abuse.	It may be an additional challenge for Adult Protective Services agencies that are already overwhelmed and underresourced.
Screening itself does not prevent harm; even if potential benefits are not clear, they are still possible.	A health care provider's perceived lack of response to screening, detection, and reporting to authorities may lead to even less screening and reporting.
Early screening leads to early detection and interventions, which may improve a victim's circumstances or stop the abuse.	Initiatives to support elder abuse awareness are encouraging, but are not great enough to justify screening.
Talking with a health care provider might be the victim's only opportunity to disclose an abusive situation.	Many current tools do not include screening for financial exploitation or neglect.

Adapted from National Center on Elder Abuse. Elder abuse screening tools for healthcare professionals. Available at: https://ncea.acl.gov/resources/docs/Research-2-Practice-Screen-Tools.pdf. Accessed August 1, 2018; and National Center on Elder Abuse. Elder abuse screening tools for healthcare professionals. Available at: http://eldermistreatment.usc.edu/wp-content/uploads/2016/10/Elder-Abuse-Screening-Tools-for-Healthcare-Professionals.pdf. Accessed August 1, 2018.

of each tool when combined [11,12]. Another screening tool, The Elder Abuse Inventory, has been widely used since the 1980s [13] and is appropriate for a variety of clinical settings. Although the tool is lengthy and has no scoring system, its use heightens an NP's awareness of potential abuse, and is available for free download at the ConsultGeri website (www.consultgeri.org) [14]. Table 2 provides detailed information on these screening tools.

Despite awareness of the need for elder abuse screening in all clinical settings, the literature has identified barriers that may prevent screening from being incorporated into routine practice [15]. NPs should be proactive in eliminating barriers that prevent them from advocating for the safety of this vulnerable patient population (Box 3).

Health care providers should be confident when approaching an elder abuse screening and assessment, while also approaching the situation with sensitivity and empathy. The victim may approach the situation with conflicting emotions, including fear of the future ("What will happen to me?"), guilt ("What if my caregiver goes to jail?"), shame ("I cannot believe I did not realize he was stealing things all this time."), and embarrassment ("Now my friends will know about it") [16]. It is important to approach the screening and/or assessment recognizing that all elder abuse victims respond differently to abuse and may not be interested in accepting assistance (Table 3).

Assessment

An elder abuse assessment typically requires a detailed history, followed by a full head-to-toe physical examination of the victim. The NP must keep in mind that multiple types of abuse often coexist. It is not the NP's job to prove abuse, but rather to accurately and thoroughly collect and document history and physical examination findings. Elder abuse is often difficult to identify, because features may mimic the normal changes of aging. Although the NP must view the physical findings in the context of multiple factors (pathophysiology, medical history, function, and mechanism of injury), there are clinical manifestations that should raise an NP's index of suspicion of abuse (Table 4) [17–19]. The patient's decisional capacity must also be assessed, because this factor may influence the type of interventions that are used in the event of abuse. It should also be noted that, during the assessment, perpetrators often refuse to allow the NP to see the older adult alone, and the history or explanation of injury does not match examination findings.

The first step in confronting a confirmed case of abuse is to ensure safety of the victim [20]. The NP should determine if there is an immediate threat of danger. Options to ensure immediate safety include calling the police department; seeking care in a shelter; emergency department or hospital admission; or respite care in a long-term care facility [20]. If there is no immediate threat, a safety plan should be created, with specific steps that the victim should take in the event a violent situation should arise.

Documentation

The NP should document all history and physical examination findings with the knowledge that the documentation may be reviewed and used in an elder

Table 2
Recommended elder abuse screening tools

Tool	No. of Items	Administration	Psychometrics	Setting	Clinical Suitability
Elder Abuse Suspicion Index	6	Administration time: 2 minutes. Completed by any health care professional to assess risk and all types of elder abuse over a 12-month period	Sensitivity: 0.77 Specificity: 0.44 Content validity in 7 diverse countries	Validated in family physicians in primary care settings	Brief tool, with an adequate ability to detect true cases of abuse, but may result in higher rate of false positive findings. A self-administered version available and is feasible, acceptable, and comprehensible
Hwalek-Sengstock Elder Abuse Screening Test	15	Administration time: 5–10 minutes. Administration by a professional or self-report. Three domains: violation of personal rights or direct abuse; characteristics of vulnerability; potentially abusive situations	Constructive and predictive validity. Weak item reliability. Good cross-cultural adaptation	Suitable for outpatient or emergency settings	Primarily assesses for domestic violence. Useful for providers who want to identify older adults with a high risk for need of protective services
Vulnerability to Abuse Screening Scale	12	Self-report of dependency, dejection, coercion, and vulnerability. 12 dichotomous questions (ie, yes/no)	Moderate ranges of reliability. Moderate to good construct validity	Not applicable	Brief, but not unreliable to assess coercion by others
Elder Abuse Inventory	42	Administration time: 12–15 minutes. Completed by health care professional. Assesses physical, social, medical, independence in older adults	Good content and construct validity. Interrater agreement. Sensitivity: 0.71; Specificity = 0.93 item reliability = 0.84; test–retest 0.83	Can be used in a variety of settings	Tool is lengthy. No scoring system

Data from Refs. [11–14]

Box 3: Barriers to elder abuse detection and reporting

Lack of training

Lack of confidence in screening ability

Lack of awareness about association between abuse and high mortality

Poor past experiences with adult protective services

Previous absence of screening tools

Disbelief that detection will lead to a solution

Fear of confrontation

Fear of compromising provider–patient relationship

Abuse signs may mimic aging changes and go unnoticed

Data from McMullen T, Schwartz K, Yaffe, M, et al. Elder abuse and its prevention: screening and detection. In: Institute of Medicine & National Research Council, editors. Elder abuse and its prevention: workshop summary. Washington (DC): The National Academies Press; 2014. p. 88–93. Available at: https://www.ncbi.nlm.nih.gov/books/NBK208569; and Schmeidel AN, Daly JM, Rosenbaum ME, et al. Healthcare professionals' perspectives on barriers to elder abuse detection and reporting in primary care settings. J Elder Abuse Negl 2012;24(1):17–36.

abuse investigation or court of law. Functional and cognitive capacity should be carefully documented to accurately illustrate the patient's abilities at the time of the examination [17]. Additionally, rather than describing the patient's report, the NP should use exact quotes ("She threatened to push me down the stairs again if I told anyone about it"). When photographing injuries, the NP should follow organization guidelines to be assured the photos may be used in an investigation. Any injury should be measured against a ruler or an object with a familiar size (quarter) to give the viewer perspective [17]. If documenting in an electronic health record that includes web access for patients and caregivers, the NP may want to place detailed notes about observations and examination findings for suspected elder abuse under a confidential section of the electronic health record or in a separate paper chart [16].

Table 3
Communication strategies

Interviewing techniques	Communication strategies	Environmental adjustments
Ask one question at a time.	Interviewer should be at eye and lip level.	Interview patient and alleged perpetrator separately.
Avoid use of leading questions.	Patient should be using all hearing and visual aids.	Conduct assessment in a private setting.
Use of respect and patience.	Interview should be at time of day when patient is most lucid.	Use good lighting.

Data from Tronetti P. Evaluating abuse in the patient with dementia. Clin Geriatr Med 2014;30(4):833–34; with permission.

Table 4
Clinical and laboratory findings commonly found in elder abuse

Medical condition	Laboratory data	Assessment findings	Causes
Alopecia	Subgalael hematoma (CT scan)	Signs of trauma to scalp	Physical abuse
Bleeding (vaginal and/or rectal)	N/A	Genital, rectal, or oral trauma—erythema, bruising, lacerations Torn, stained, or bloody undergarments	Sexual abuse
Bruising	N/A	Atypical locations (not over bony prominences)— lateral arms, head and neck region, posterior torso, buttocks, genitalia, soles of feet Bruising associated with elder abuse are usually large (>5 cm) and present on the face, lateral right arm, and posterior torso Color and duration of bruising are not reliable indicators of intentional injury Symmetric injuries Unexplained injuries Bruising around breasts or genitals Unsuitable clothing for season (to cover up bruising)	Intent to harm (physical abuse) Sexual abuse
Burns and lacerations	N/A	Burn in stocking/glove pattern (suggests forced immersion) or cigarette pattern Wrist and/or ankle lesions or scars (suggesting inappropriate restraints)	Physical abuse 40%–70% of burns are related to elder abuse Burn patterns in elder abuse resemble those found in child abuse Lacerations more likely to occur as a result of blunt force trauma, restraints, friction Abrasions retain the form of the device used to create the trauma

Condition	Labs/Tests	Clinical Signs	Associated Abuse Type
Contractures	N/A	Poor hygiene Intertriginal dermatitis Presence of lice, scabies	Neglect
Dehydration	↑ Sodium ↑BUN/creatinine ratio >20 ↑ Uric acid ↑ Hbg/HCT	Poor skin turgor Fecal impaction Dry mucus membranes Sunken eyes Orthostatic hypotension Tachycardia	Neglect: withholding fluids, avoid fluid intake to ↓ urinary incontinence, avoidance of need to provide care
Depression and anxiety	N/A	Sucking, rocking, mumbling to self Emotional withdrawal	All abuse types
Fracture (occult)	N/A	Fracture pattern that does not stem from direction of a fall	Physical abuse Fracture in nonambulatory patient is suspicious for abuse
Hyper/hypothermia	↑ Serum CK Abnormal thyroid function tests	Elevated body temperature Sepsis Dehydration	Neglect: lack of air conditioner or heat, excessive or inadequate clothing Neglect and/or physical abuse: neuroleptic malignant syndrome (hyperthermia: related to overuse of neuroleptic medications)
Infection	Recurrent UTI Aspiration pneumonia Unexplained sexually transmitted illnesses Infected pressure injuries	Urinary frequency or burning Vaginal discharge Recurrent choking with feeding Advanced stage pressure injuries with signs of infection or poor care	Sexual abuse Physical abuse: Force feeding Neglect: not providing adequate personal hygiene, turning in bed, or nutrition
Malnutrition	↓ Serum albumin ↓ Serum prealbumin ↓ Transferrin ↓ Cholesterol ↓ Total lymphocyte count Anemia	BMI <21 kg/m² Triceps skin fold, 80% normal Muscle wasting Functional decline	Financial abuse (inability to purchase food) Neglect: withholding food, unattended dental issues, poor feeding techniques for dysphagia, inattention to food preferences

(continued on next page)

Table 4
(continued)

Medical condition	Laboratory data	Assessment findings	Causes
Moisture-associated skin damage	N/A	Dermatitis in perineal area (related to prolonged exposure to urine and stool) Patient wearing multiple briefs Scratch marks on skin	Neglect
Ophthalmic hemorrhages	N/A	Subconjunctival, vitreous, or retinal hemorrhages with evidence of head trauma	Physical abuse
Pressure injuries	N/A	Skin breakdown to perineal area in patient with urinary and fecal incontinence or over bony prominences Dried feces and urine imbedded in wound Old dressing in place	Neglect
Rhabdomyolysis	↑ Serum CK + Urine myoglobin ↑Sodium ↓Phosphate ↓potassium Acute renal insufficiency	Signs of bruising/falling Signs of wrist/ankle restraints Signs of malnutrition and dehydration Hypo/hyperthermia	Physical abuse: trauma—muscle injury Neglect: prolonged immobility secondary to restraints, severe malnutrition and dehydration, lack of air conditioning/heat causing hypo/hyperthermia (overuse or misuse of neuroleptics)
Toxicology	Blood/hair samples: presence of recreational or prescription drugs or toxins not prescribed to the patient (ETOH, THC, LSD, amphetamines, narcotics, sedatives/hypnotics)	Sedation Somnolence Euphoria Cognitive impairment Depression Cardiovascular events	Inappropriate administration of medication with intent to chemically restrain Intention to harm

Abbreviations: BMI, body mass index; BUN, blood urea nitrogen; CK, creatine kinase; CT, computed tomography; ETOH, ethyl alcohol; HCT, hematocrit; Hgb, hemoglobin; N/A, not applicable; UTI, urinary tract infection.
Data from Refs. [17–19]

COMMUNITY RESOURCES

The majority of elder abuse victims endure their situation in isolation and do not use formal resources. Formal resources are important as they hold perpetrators responsible for their actions and reduce the risk of revictimization [21]. Formal support services include law enforcement, adult protective services, and other community-based response programs; informal support services include support from friends and family members [5,22,23]. Coordinated community support via interagency collaboration (law enforcement, social services, APS, and mental health and medical agencies) is a relatively new recommended strategy to effectively respond to elder abuse. Many community services and resources receive federal funding and support. Additionally, these support services may also provide preventative measures for elder abuse (Box 4).

PREVENTION

The adequate prevention of elder abuse involves interventions from multiple sectors of society. Although prevention interventions have been presented, no systematic research has been done to measure and evaluate their effects [24]. Sixteen elder

Box 4: National elder abuse support services and resources

Organization	Resource(s) provided
Adult Protective Services (http://www.napsa-now.org/)	Investigation of abuse allegations; assessment of individual's safety and need for assistance. Determine what services would be beneficial to maintain safety, health, and independence.
National Center on Elder Abuse (https://ncea.acl.gov/)	Reports, webinars, podcasts, and databases. Website provides links to state-specific information, advance planning tools.
Long Term Care Ombudsman (http://www.theconsumervoice.org/)	Works to resolve complaints made by or on behalf of residents in long-term care facilities.
Family Justice Center Alliance (https://www.familyjusticecenter.org/)	Provides technical assistance, resources, and training for funded centers and nonfunded Centers and multidisciplinary teams who do not receive federal funding. Helps communities to plan, start, operate, and expand Family Justice Centers and similar multiagency service models.
Elder Consumer Protection Program at Stetson University College of Law Center for Excellence in Elder Law (https://www.stetson.edu/law/academics/elder/ecpp/)	General and legal matters regarding elder consumer fraud protection and awareness.
Area Agency on Aging (https://www.n4a.org/)	Provides services including home-delivered meals, legal assistance, and referrals
National Council on Aging (https://www.ncoa.org/)	Services (education, technical assistance) depend on location.

abuse intervention studies have been conducted, most of which have focused on an education intervention for the caregiver [24]. Tenets of successful child abuse prevention programs have also been translated into elder abuse prevention strategies [25]. Other prevention strategies that have been tested include support groups for caregivers and daily money management to hinder financial exploitation [24].

In 2018, the Barbara and Richard Csomay Center for Gerontological Excellence at the University of Iowa College of Nursing published elder abuse prevention guidelines. The domains of prevention include formal and informal prevention measures. Although some elder abuse prevention interventions studies have been conducted, no systematic research has measured and evaluated the effects of these interventions (Box 5).

IMPLICATIONS FOR PRACTICE

With the growing number of older adults accessing health care in the outpatient setting, it is prudent that NPs be knowledgeable of risk factors and clinical signs/

Box 5: Intervention strategies for elder abuse prevention

Domain	Intervention
Legislation	Mandatory reporting of abuse or suspected abuse
	States with mandatory reporting laws have significantly higher investigation rates
	Elder abuse definitions in state regulations
	The greater the number of elder abuse definitions in state regulations, the higher the substantiation rates and substantiation/investigations ratios
	Adult protective services caseworkers work exclusively with elder abuse
	Higher substantiation/investigation ratios than caseworkers assigned to investigate both child and elder abuse
	Tracking reports of abuse
	Leads to higher investigation and substantiation rates as well as substantiation/investigation ratios
Education	Health Professionals:
	The Elder Investment Fraud and Financial Exploitation Prevention Program provides training on identifying abuse, how to refer at-risk patients to State Securities Regulators or APS
	Bank employees
	OWN IT Model (Wells Fargo Bank): training to raise awareness and empower them to act when exploitation is suspected
	Training professionals across professions and occupations (first responders, service providers, lawyers, postal workers, home-delivered meals, door persons, staff in institutions)

(continued on next page)

(continued)	
Domain	Intervention
Caregiver support/ caregiver respite	No studies have shown that respite decreases or prevents elder abuse
	Three types of respite: adult day services, in-home, and institutional
	Types of caregiver support needed: instrumental, informational, emotional
	Resources for Enhancing Alzheimer's Caregiver Health
	Focus on problem-solving techniques and development of written action plans
	The New York University Caregiver Intervention
	Individual/family counseling, support groups, continuous availability of counselors
Social support	Not tested as an intervention to prevent elder abuse
	Social support through community integration (ie, better access to public transportation)
	Emergency shelters: Collaborative model using existing resource of community. Involves the use of a congregate or institutional living setting (ie, nursing home) that can be used to shelter, protect and empower victims of elder abuse
	Eliciting Change in At-Risk Elders program
	Community partnerships with law enforcement and program staff at community assistance program for seniors
Batterer interventions	Marginally effective in preventing elder abuse
	Cognitive–behavioral therapy: Focus on changing person's thinking and associated depression-related behaviors
Money management programs	Technology-based programs (smart phone applications for tracking financial fraud)
	Daily money management programs
	Services to assist individuals who have difficulty managing money
	Offered via older adult assistance agencies or area agency on aging/protective service agencies
	Individuals associated with the American Association of Daily Money Managers are reputable (https://www.aadmm.com)
Multidisciplinary teams	Interagency collaboration: Legal services, shelters, victim protection, educators, service providers
	Elder Abuse Forensic Centers
	Case has 10 times greater likelihood of being presented to the district attorney
Circle of friends	Group of individuals who share a common interest

Data from Refs.[12,24,25]

symptoms of elder abuse. Familiarity with screening tests will aid NPs, should the need arise for a more thorough investigation. The patient–NP relationship should be one of mutual trust that fosters an environment conducive to honest conversations about any threats to one's safety and well-being. When such situations are handled with sensitivity, the patient is more likely to share details of abuse. Victims should understand they are not at fault for their abuse and there are resources available to mitigate future abuse. The NP should be transparent with a patient about concerns for abuse and should be forthright about any referral that will be made to law enforcement or an APS agency. NPs can make a positive impact on the eradication of elder abuse in their primary care practices.

References

[1] US Census Bureau. American fact finder. Available at: https://factfinder.census.gov/faces/nav/jsf/pages/index.xhtml. Accessed August 13, 2018.

[2] Ortman JM, Velkoff VA, Hogan H. An aging nation: the older population in the United States. Washington, DC: U.S. Census Bureau; 2014. p. 1–28. Available at: http://www.bowchair.com/uploads/9/8/4/9/98495722/agingcensus.pdf. Accessed August 13, 2018.

[3] World Health Organization. Elder abuse. Available at: http://www.who.int/ageing/projects/elder_abuse/en/. Accessed August 13, 2018.

[4] Centers for Disease Control and Prevention. Elder abuse: definitions. Available at: https://www.cdc.gov/violenceprevention/elderabuse/definitions.html. Accessed August 30, 2018.

[5] Acierno R, Hernandez MA, Amstadter AB, et al. Prevalence and correlates of emotional, physical, sexual, and financial abuse and potential neglect in the United States: the national elder mistreatment study. Am J Public Health 2010;100:292–7.

[6] Yon Y, Mikton CR, Gassoumis ZD, et al. Elder abuse prevalence in community settings: a systematic review and meta-analysis. Lancet 2017;5(2):e147–56.

[7] Dong XQ. Elder abuse: systematic review and implications for practice. J Am Geriatr Soc 2015;63(6):1214–38.

[8] Johannesen M, LoGiudice D. Elder abuse: a systematic review of risk factors in community-dwelling elders. Age Ageing 2013;42:292–8.

[9] The United States Dept of Justice. State elder abuse statutes. Available at: https://www.justice.gov/elderjustice/elder-justice-statutes-0#SL3. Accessed August 13, 2018.

[10] National Center on Elder Abuse. Elder abuse screening tools for healthcare professionals. Available at: http://eldermistreatment.usc.edu/wp-content/uploads/2016/10/Elder-Abuse-Screening-Tools-for-Healthcare-Professionals.pdf. Accessed August 1, 2018.

[11] Burnett J, Achenbaum WA, Murphy KP. Prevention and early identification of elder abuse. Clin Geriatr Med 2014;30(4):743–59.

[12] McMullen T, Schwartz K, Yaffe M, et al. Elder abuse and its prevention: screening and detection. In: Institute of Medicine & National Research Council, editor. Elder abuse and its prevention: workshop summary. Washington (DC): The National Academies Press; 2014. p. 88–93. Available at: https://www.ncbi.nlm.nih.gov/books/NBK208569/.

[13] Gallione C, Dal Molin A, Cristina FV, et al. Screening tools for the identification of elder abuse: a systematic review. J Clin Nurs 2017;26:2154–76.

[14] ConsultGeri. Elder mistreatment and abuse. Available at: www.consultgeri.org/geriatric-topics/elder-mistreatment-and-abuse. Accessed August 1, 2018.

[15] Schmeidel AN, Daly JM, Rosenbaum ME, et al. Healthcare professionals' perspectives on barriers to elder abuse detection and reporting in primary care settings. J Elder Abuse Negl 2012;24(1):17–36.

[16] Tronetti P. Evaluating abuse in the patient with dementia. Clin Geriatr Med 2014;30(4):825–38.

[17] Gibbs LM. Understanding the medical markers of elder abuse and neglect: physical examination findings. Clin Geriatr Med 2014;30(4):687–712.

[18] LoFaso VM, Rosen T. Medical and laboratory indicators of elder abuse and neglect. Clin Geriatr Med 2014;30(4):713–28.

[19] Rosen A, Alyssa E, Fulmer T. Recognizing mistreatment in older adults. In: Fulmer T, Chernof B, editors. Handbook of geriatric assessment. 5th edition. Burlington (MA): Jones & Bartlett Learning; 2019. p. 215–30.

[20] Lachs M, Rosen T. Elder mistreatment. In: Halter JB, Ouslander JG, Studenski S, et al, editors. Hazzard's geriatric medicine and gerontology. 7th edition. Columbus (OH): McGraw-Hill Education; 2017. p. 821–30.

[21] Burnes D, Breckman R, Henderson CR, et al. Utilization of formal support services for elder abuse: do informal supporters make a difference? Gerontologist 2018;21; https://doi.org/10.1093/geront/gny074.

[22] Amstadter AB, Cisler JM, McCauley JL, et al. Do incident and perpetrator characteristics of elder mistreatment differ by gender of the victim? results from the national elder mistreatment study. J Elder Abuse Negl 2011;23(1):43–57.

[23] Lachs MS, Berman J. Under the radar: New York State elder abuse prevalence study. New York: William B. Hoyt Memorial New York State Children, Family Trust Fund, New York State Office of Children and Family Service; 2011.

[24] Daly JM, Butcher HK. Evidence-based practice guideline: elder abuse prevention. J Gerontol Nurs 2018;44(7):21–30.

[25] Teresi JA, Burnes D, Skowron MA, et al. State-of-the-science on prevention of elder abuse and lessons learned from child abuse and domestic violence prevention: toward a conceptual framework for research. J Elder Abuse Negl 2016;28(4–5):263–300.

Women's Health

Advances in Family Practice Nursing 1 (2019) 117–129

ADVANCES IN FAMILY PRACTICE NURSING

ELSEVIER
MOSBY

First-trimester Bleeding
Assessment, Diagnosis, and Management
by the Primary Care Nurse Practitioner

Check for updates

Elizabeth Munoz, CNM, MSN*,
Heather Robbins, DNP, MBA, RN

Vanderbilt University School of Nursing, 461 21st Avenue South, Nashville, TN 37240, USA

Keywords
- Vaginal bleeding • Miscarriage • Spontaneous abortion • Ultrasound
- First-trimester bleeding • Pregnancy • History • Assessment

Key points
- Bleeding within the first 14 weeks is common and often associated with anxiety, causing women to seek evaluation by a health care provider.
- Many women do not establish prenatal care until late in the first trimester but seek medical care when early pregnancy bleeding occurs, offering the opportunity for primary nurse practitioners to provide this care.
- Primary care nurse practitioners are qualified to provide services, such as physical assessment and ordering of diagnostics (laboratory tests and radiology) that aid in assessing, diagnosing, and treating first-trimester bleeding.
- Additionally, the primary care nurse practitioner refers patients to the appropriate level of care or expedite emergency care, if indicated.

INTRODUCTION

Many women experience bleeding in the first trimester of pregnancy and may seek care from their primary providers prior to the initiation of obstetric care. Often, obstetric providers do not offer a new patient pregnancy visit until later in the first trimester, and primary care nurse practitioners (NPs) may be asked by their patients to help during this time, especially when there is

---

Special Statement by Authors: Within this article, the pronoun she and the nouns woman/women are used to discuss first-trimester bleeding in pregnancy. The authors support gender-affirming language and encourage individualized care with client-preferred pronouns.

*Corresponding author. *E-mail address:* elizabeth.g.munoz@vumc.org

https://doi.org/10.1016/j.yfpn.2019.01.006

the concern of first-trimester bleeding. With the exception of acute hemorrhage (where a patient needs to be seen in the emergency department), the initial assessment and evaluation of first-trimester bleeding can be provided within a clinic setting. The reported bleeding could be vaginal, cervical, or uterine and locating the origin of the bleeding by performing a full examination is a key step in achieving an accurate diagnosis [1]. Many providers move directly to obtaining a transvaginal ultrasound but this is not always the most effective way to gather the needed evidence. By starting with a thorough patient history and physical examination, for example, an NP can rule out bleeding from a cervical polyp, vaginal infection, or labial lesion. The provider may even see evidence of the products of conception in the cervix or the vagina during examination with a speculum, which would diagnose a spontaneous abortion (SAB) clearly without necessitating imaging and, thus, avoiding cost to the patient.

Through the use of a thorough history, physical examination, laboratory assessment, and imaging, there are many opportunities for primary care providers to recognize, diagnose, and treat women who present with vaginal bleeding in early pregnancy. Therefore, it is imperative that primary care clinicians be able to recognize and diagnose early pregnancy warning signs. In the following paragraphs, a step-by-step guide is offered for thoughtfully diagnosing the cause of bleeding in early pregnancy.

HISTORY

Early pregnancy is a time of rapid, complex embryonic and fetal development. Symptoms can occur early in a pregnancy that initiate concern and cause women to present to their provider for evaluation. One of the symptoms that often cause alarm and distress for a patient is vaginal bleeding. First-trimester bleeding is defined as bleeding that occurs from 0 to 13 weeks and 6 days and is commonly experienced in pregnancy. Approximately 25% of all women with a known pregnancy experience first-trimester bleeding [2,3]. The amount of bleeding experienced by women can range from light spotting to heavy and menstrual-like in quantity and can be either painless or accompanied by painful cramps. Up to three-quarters of patients who have bleeding report light spotting for several days [4]. Bleeding in the first trimester can be a benign, normal variant of pregnancy or it can represent more serious complications. The most common cause of first-trimester bleeding is threatened miscarriage [5]. According to Knez and colleagues [6] and Tamizzian and Arulkumaran [7], 50% of pregnancies complicated by bleeding may progress normally, whereas the remaining 50% of pregnancies may experience pregnancy loss.

Other common causes for early bleeding in pregnancy are

- Implantation bleeding
- Cervical polyp
- Maternal clotting disorders

- Placental complications
- Bacterial vaginosis
- Genital infections, such as gonorrhea and chlamydia [5]

ASSESSMENT

Assessment of a patient presenting with complaints of first-trimester bleeding encompasses steps that help guide providers to an appropriate diagnosis and treatment plan. After it has been determined that a patient can be safely assessed in the clinic, the next steps include several categories of thorough assessment techniques to provide a complete and accurate evaluation. Watkins and colleagues [2] identified 4 major assessment and evaluation components that help in this process.

The following illustrates the major assessment categories and key elements essential to performing an accurate assessment on a patient presenting with first-trimester bleeding.

Conducting a thorough patient history is one of the most important tools in understanding and diagnosing first-trimester bleeding. Factors to explore when taking a patient history include 13 key variables (Fig. 1). Questions associated with bleeding should help providers understand the frequency, amount, and color of blood. Associated symptoms and warning signs may include dizziness, nausea, fever, and pelvic, abdominal, and lower back pain [5]. It is important to know if a patient's pregnancy has been confirmed, when it was confirmed, and by what method (quantitative vs qualitative). If known, last menstrual period (LMP) indicates how far along the pregnancy is in gestational weeks (estimated gestational

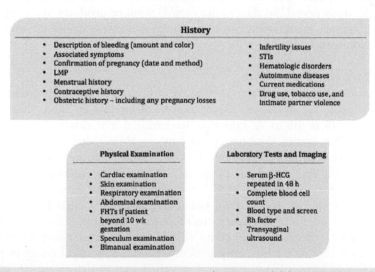

Fig. 1. Assessment components, examination elements, and laboratory testing for first-trimester bleeding. FHT, fetal heart tones; STI, sexually transmitted infection.

age) and provides an estimated due date, which are variables important for diagnosis and treatment. Obtaining menstrual, contraceptive, obstetric, and sexually transmitted infection histories aids providers in determining if there is any underlying gynecologic pathology or concern for future infertility. Special attention should be given to patient or family history of hematologic disorders and autoimmune disorders because these disease processes can cause abnormal bleeding profiles [2]. As with any patient history, current medications should be reconciled, identifying any medications that are cause for concern during pregnancy. Social history should include questions about illicit drug use, alcohol use, tobacco use, intimate partner violence, if the pregnancy is desired, and social support [2].

Physical examination

In addition to vital signs, a focused physical examination that includes several key systems provides clues for the cause of bleeding and helps clinicians evaluate the overall health of patients and pregnancies. The respiratory and cardiac systems should be evaluated for abnormalities, such as tachycardia, murmurs, tachypnea, and shortness of breath. The integumentary system should be evaluated for abnormalities such as diffuse ecchymosis and petechiae which could indicate bleeding disorders [2]. Pain or tenderness upon palpation during an abdominal examination raises suspicion for a ruptured ectopic pregnancy or intra-abdominal bleeding. It is appropriate to attempt auscultation of fetal heart tones with a Doppler device if the pregnancy is at least 10 weeks' gestation [2]. A vaginal examination should be performed and should include speculum and bimanual examinations. The speculum examination may reveal bleeding in the vaginal vault or products of conception, and a bimanual examination can be performed to assess size of the uterus in correlation with LMP [2,5].

Laboratory tests and imaging

If not done already, a serum quantitative β-human chorionic gonadotropin (β-hCG) may be drawn as confirmation of pregnancy and should be repeated in 48 hours to 72 hours to determine if it is rising appropriately. A β-hCG that is not doubling or is low or slow rising may indicate a nonviable or ectopic pregnancy. If the result is more than doubling and increasing sharply, molar pregnancy should be considered. There are wide ranges for acceptable β-hCG levels depending on gestational age (See American Pregnancy Association, Guideline to HCG Levels During Pregnancy: http://americanpregnancy.org/while-pregnant/hcg-levels/) [8]. Additionally, a complete blood cell count should be drawn to assess for anemia related to excess blood loss. Any patient who has vaginal bleeding in pregnancy should have a blood type and screen drawn to determine Rh status. If the woman is Rh-negative, she should receive $Rh_o(D)$ immunoglobulin within 48 hours to 72 hours after the onset of bleeding. Ultimately, imaging using a transvaginal ultrasound may be warranted to help determine viability and dating of the pregnancy as well as other possible causes of bleeding [2].

Differential diagnosis

There are multiple reasons vaginal bleeding occurs during the early weeks of pregnancy, ranging from normal or common to serious and/or emergent. Less worrisome causes of bleeding include cervical polyps, bleeding from the ovarian follicle from which ovulation occurred (corpus luteal cyst), implantation bleeding and retrochorionic hemorrhage, and bleeding between the fetal membrane sac and the uterine wall [2]. These less serious differential diagnoses often do not require any urgent medical treatment, although it is important to communicate to patients that as many as 50% of those experiencing signs of a threatened abortion could lead to miscarriage [2]. Higher-acuity possible causes of vaginal bleeding in the first-trimester include miscarriage (threatened or missed), ectopic pregnancy, and molar pregnancy. Table 1 guides the practitioner through the various differential diagnoses, including patient education points and signs for when a patient needs to be referred to the emergency department.

DIAGNOSIS

The presence of vaginal bleeding in early pregnancy is not always an emergency nor does it confirm that there has been a miscarriage. For example, the provider must consider the amount of bleeding present and if the patient is hemodynamically stable. Once a diagnosis has been determined based on symptoms, the client should be counseled on treatment options, including in some cases (such as an uncomplicated spontaneous abortion) the option for expectant management. The following sections address the diagnosis, treatment, and management of differing scenarios that can occur when a client presents with first-trimester bleeding.

TREATMENT

The treatment and management of patients in the first trimester of pregnancy presenting to a primary care provider's office with vaginal bleeding are guided by the diagnosis or suspected diagnosis associated with bleeding. A majority of patients evaluated may be safely managed in the outpatient setting with close follow-up. In many cases, the exact etiology of early pregnancy bleeding remains undiagnosed despite thorough evaluation. To reduce morbidity and mortality associated with ruptured ectopic pregnancy, hemorrhage, and significant pelvic infection (septic abortion or pelvic inflammatory disease), however, it is important that the primary care provider identifies these conditions in a timely manner. Patients with hemodynamic instability, peritoneal signs (rebound tenderness, tenderness to percussion, and abdominal guarding), or hemorrhage should be transferred to the emergency department to expedite treatment. Non–pregnancy-related (traumatic, infectious, malignant, inflammatory, and structural) diagnoses should be treated appropriately, with special attention to pregnancy considerations, should a pregnancy be ongoing.

Table 1
Differential diagnoses of first-trimester bleeding

Differential diagnosis	Common symptoms	Diagnostic steps	Treatment options and patient education
Cervical polyp	Random vaginal bleeding Postcoital bleeding Bleeding heavily with papanicolaou test	Pelvic examination in clinic with speculum examination to visualize the presence of polyp	Leave in situ or referral for removal of polyp
Hemorrhagic corpus luteum, also known as bleeding from the site of ovulation within the ovary	Bleeding at random in the first few weeks of pregnancy	+UPT Verify that blood is coming from cervical os (the cervical opening) on pelvic examination or vaginal bleeding reported by patient Pelvic ultrasound to confirm	None indicated No reason for pelvic rest
Subchorionic hemorrhage	Bleeding occurs between the fetal sac membrane and the uterine wall	+UPT Verify bleeding on pelvic examination Pelvic ultrasound to confirm	May consider pelvic rest if bleeding continues Plan follow-up ultrasound to ensure stability/resolution
Vaginal abrasion	Postcoital bleeding Patient reports vaginal irritation Scant bleeding; blood may appear more brown than bright red	+UPT Verify bleeding is not coming from cervical os on pelvic examination Visualize area of bleeding to confirm no lesion present	Can avoid IC until bleeding event subsides

Abbreviations: IC, intercourse; UPT, positive urine pregnancy test.

It is standard of care in the United States that $Rh_o(D)$ immunoglobulin be administered within 72 hours of vaginal bleeding in previously unsensitized patients with negative Rh factor, to prevent $Rh_o(D)$ alloimmunization and its sequelae for the fetus. A dose of 50 µg is adequate for first-trimester bleeding; however, product availability is usually limited to a standard 300 µg, which is routinely used in this setting.

Viable intrauterine pregnancy

If transvaginal ultrasound demonstrates a viable intrauterine pregnancy, a diagnosis of threatened abortion should be made. The patient should be counseled that a majority of pregnancies complicated by early vaginal bleeding continue to viability [9–12]. Moderate or heavy vaginal bleeding (similar to or heavier than a menses) is associated with miscarriage in approximately 24% of these pregnancies, a rate of approximately 2.6 of those with light bleeding [9]. Short-interval follow-up of a patient with threatened abortion is prudent, and follow-up β-hCG levels and ultrasound may be indicated.

Women often seek guidance on restrictions or interventions that may positively influence the outcome of a desired pregnancy at this time. There is no evidence that any intervention lowers the risk of progression of a threatened abortion to a spontaneous abortion; therefore, pelvic rest, supplements, medications, or any other interventions for this specific purpose are not recommended [13–15]. Medical comorbidities and modifiable risk factors, should they exist, should be considered within clinical context and addressed appropriately.

Nonviable intrauterine pregnancy

Nonviable pregnancies include anembryonic gestation, embryonic demise, and incomplete abortions. These pregnancies may be managed expectantly, medically, or surgically. Options for management in stable and uncomplicated patients should be driven by patient preference, because they have all been demonstrated to be safe and efficacious [16–18]. Women with persistent, heavy vaginal bleeding, with signs of hemodynamic instability or infection should be managed surgically to expedite complete evacuation of uterine contents. An excellent patient education handout reviewing management options with considerations and common questions is available from the Reproductive Health Access Project, which is freely accessible on their Web site.

Expectant management

Clinically stable women without signs of infection may choose to await spontaneous passage of products of conception. Based on prospective observational studies, a majority of women, 70% to 84%, experience a complete, spontaneous miscarriage within 2 weeks of the diagnosis of a nonviable pregnancy [19,20]. Efficacy is higher in incomplete abortion and decreases with missed abortion and anembryonic gestations [19,20]. Routine antibiotics are not necessary or recommended. Expectant management may be observed for as long as a woman remains stable and without signs or symptoms of infection.

- Counseling should include the following:
  - Spontaneous passage of products of conception can take 8 weeks or more, although a majority of women experience complete miscarriage within 2 weeks.
  - Bleeding is likely to begin as light; progress to bright red with moderate to heavy flow, with cramping and clotting, which may last approximately 4 hours; and then taper. Lighter bleeding for 1 week to 2 weeks following a spontaneous abortion is possible and may start and stop a few times.
  - Patient education should include bleeding and infection precautions and include how to contact the on-call provider after hours.

- ○ Change in management type may be opted for at any time.
- Office follow-up should be dependent on course; however, with report of bleeding consistent with passage of products of conception, a 1-week to 2-week visit thereafter allows for a follow-up β-hCG level or transvaginal ultrasound, if indicated, and space and time for questions, concerns, and emotional processing.
- Expectant management may be observed for as long as the patient remains stable, without signs of infection, and may take 8 weeks or more for resolution.
- Should the patient desire to change management types, the option to change to either medical or surgical management should be offered at any time.

Medical management

Although recent data have demonstrated the superiority of administration of mifepristone (progesterone receptor antagonist) prior to misoprostol (prostaglandin analog) compared with misoprostol alone for the medical management of first-trimester nonviable pregnancies [21], access to mifepristone due to Food and Drug Administration regulations is significantly limited and it is not sold in retail pharmacies. It cannot be prescribed to patients directly and can be dispensed only by a clinician who meets manufacturer-specific requirements and is trained and approved by the manufacturer program. For primary care nurse-practitioners, it is not currently routinely used in clinical practice; however, if local specialty clinics are available, referral to a women's health practice that stocks mifepristone in house may be warranted.

Misoprostol is a synthetic prostaglandin E1 compound, which, in the setting of uterine evacuation, works primarily via induction of uterine contractions but has secondary effects of cervical softening and dilation. It is available in the United States in generic and brand forms. Although multiple protocols exist [22], the American College of Obstetricians and Gynecologists recommends an initial dose of 800 μg, placed vaginally, and repeated no earlier than 3 hours and typically within 7 days if the first dose fails to produce complete expulsion [23]. In most cases, women experience moderate to significant cramping and vaginal bleeding with clotting similar to a heavy menses, which lasts between 2 hours and 6 hours. Continued vaginal bleeding for 7 days to 14 days, in a light to moderate fashion, can be expected. Prescriptions or instructions for over-the-counter analgesics should be provided. For most undergoing medical management, an opioid is not necessary for pain relief and is not routinely recommended. Side effects with vaginal dosing are attenuated; however, nausea, vomiting, chills, and diarrhea are possible. Oral or buccal dosing increases the incidence and severity of these side effects; an antiemetic in these cases is warranted [24].

Surgical management

Uterine evacuation via manual vacuum aspiration, vacuum curettage, or sharp curettage is a safe and effective method of resolving a nonviable pregnancy in the first trimester [25]. This procedure is performed by women's health providers only and, most commonly, by obstetrics-gynecology physicians. Manual vacuum aspiration is usually performed in the office setting under local anesthesia. Vacuum curettage and sharp curettage are typically performed in ambulatory surgery centers or hospital operating rooms. Benefits to surgical management include faster time to resolution of a nonviable pregnancy, because the procedure typically takes 10 minutes to 20 minutes, with an efficacy rate greater than or equal to medical management [26]. Additionally, need for follow-up office visits, ultrasounds, and unplanned hospital visits are likely less than with expectant and medical management [27]. Women with hemodynamic instability or signs or symptoms of infection should be directed to the emergency room for further evaluation and management. Stable patients can be referred on a routine or urgent outpatient basis, depending on the clinical scenario. A patient education handout giving anticipatory guidance on what to expect with a manual vacuum aspiration can be found at the Web site for the Reproductive Health Access Project.

Ectopic, gestational trophoblastic disease

Ectopic pregnancy is fairly rare, with an incidence rate of approximately 0.64%, but a diagnosis that should be considered in any pregnancy to prevent associated maternal morbidity and mortality [28]. More than 90% of ectopic pregnancies are located within the uterine tubes [29]. Options for treatment in this population include both medical (with methotrexate therapy [folate inhibitor]) and surgical (via salpingostomy or salpingectomy). Medical treatment may be considered in stable patients with a confirmed unruptured ectopic pregnancy and in whom methotrexate is not contraindicated [30]. Surgical management is indicated in unstable patients with signs or symptoms concerning for a ruptured mass. In these cases, further evaluation in an emergent setting is likely warranted. With stable patients cared for in settings with adequate access to a women's health provider with specialization in managing ectopic pregnancies, it is recommended an urgent referral be made. Discussion of management of ectopic pregnancies is beyond the scope of this article; however, evidence-based resources are available elsewhere.

Care after an early pregnancy loss

Office follow-up after resolution of a nonviable pregnancy should include

- Assessment for acute blood loss anemia
- Contraceptive counseling versus preconception counseling
- Recommendations for referral to a maternal fetal medicine, fertility specialist, and genetics counselor should pregnancy loss be recurrent (≥3 consecutive pregnancies)
- Assessment for need for psychosocial referrals, including therapist/grief support group

- Appendix 1 can be used as a worksheet to track and coordinate follow-up for patients experiencing SAB symptoms.

A study published in 2015 suggests that many misconceptions regarding early pregnancy loss are common [31]. As such, it is important to review that miscarriage is common, affecting up to 20% of known pregnancies, and in greater than 50% of cases is caused by chromosomal abnormalities in the embryo/fetus. It is not uncommon for women to express feelings of guilt, shame, and loneliness or a feeling that they could have prevented the loss [31]. Patients should be reassured that exercise, heavy lifting, stress, past sexually transmitted infections, past contraceptive use, and past abortions are not associated with early pregnancy loss.

As within any clinical setting, religious and cultural awareness and culturally appropriate care are highly relevant to providing excellent care. Some religions and cultures may experience early pregnancy loss similar to the loss of a child [31]. NPs are uniquely adept at providing holistic, compassionate, supportive care to patients and their families during this time.

HEALTH PROMOTION

Health promotion related to first-trimester bleeding is multifactorial and depends on the cause of bleeding, diagnosis, and whether a pregnancy is viable or nonviable. If the pregnancy is found viable and the client desires to continue the pregnancy, reassurance and guidance for expectations concerning the remainder of the pregnancy should be discussed [32,33]. As the pregnancy progresses, thorough discussion of concerns, such as abnormal bleeding and pain, should be outlined for the patient specific to each trimester. If the patient does not desire to remain pregnant and the pregnancy is viable, she should be referred to the appropriate provider for pregnancy options counseling as soon as possible.

If the pregnancy is determined nonviable, discussion surrounding treatment options and management of a miscarriage should occur. Research shows that the risk of miscarriage increases with age. One SAB does not increase a woman's risk of a second SAB [5]. If a woman has had recurrent miscarriages, however, the risk of another miscarriage is increased by up to 50% and an infertility work-up with a specialist may be offered [5]. Additionally, the patient may benefit from referral to a hematologist or endocrinologist, and additional tests may be evaluated to determine if there are underlying conditions that would cause bleeding during pregnancy or pregnancy loss [32]. Ultimately, health promotion efforts for a woman experiencing bleeding in early pregnancy should be patient centered and therapeutic, providing support and reassurance appropriate for the situation.

SUMMARY

Bleeding in early pregnancy is a common occurrence, and providing care for a client experiencing first-trimester bleeding can be intimidating for providers who do not regularly care for pregnant women. Not all women who present with this type of bleeding go on to experience a miscarriage, although miscarriage occurs somewhat frequently. The primary care provider may be tasked with assessing and diagnosing miscarriage and other complications, such as ectopic and molar pregnancies, prior to the pregnant woman seeing an obstetrics provider. Using the tools provided in this article, the primary care NP can feel more confident in assessing for complications, which may require emergency care versus an uncomplicated spontaneous abortion or nonobstetric cause of vaginal bleeding in pregnancy.

Acknowledgments

The authors wish to acknowledge contributions to this article by Nicole Mercer, MSN, CNM, FNP-C.

References

[1] Committee on Practice Bulletins—Gynecology. Early pregnancy loss. Practice Bulletin No. 150. American College of Obstetricians and Gynecologists. Obstet Gynecol 2015;125: 1258–67.

[2] Watkins EJ, Hellams A, Saldanha C. Caring for a patient with first-trimester bleeding. JAAPA 2017;30(6):15–20.

[3] Available at: www.reproductiveaccess.org/wp-content/uploads/2014/10/2017-11-EPL-algorithm.pdf. Accessed on August 25, 2018.

[4] Cohain JS. First trimester bleeding is common. Midwifery Today 2017;123:52–3.

[5] Thortensen KA. Midwifery management of first trimester bleeding and early pregnancy loss. J Midwifery Womens Health 2000;45(6):481–92.

[6] Knez J, Day A, Jurkovic D. Ultrasound imaging in the management of bleeding and pain in early pregnancy. Best Pract Res Clin Obstet Gynaecol 2014;28(5):621–36.

[7] Tamizian O, Arulkumaran S. Bleeding in early pregnancy. Curr Obstet Gynaecol 2001;11: 70–7.

[8] American Pregnancy Association. Human Chorionic Gonadotropin (HCG): the pregnancy hormone. Available at: http://americanpregnancy.org/while-pregnant/hcg-levels/. Accessed October 31, 2018.

[9] Poulose T, Richardson R, Ewings P, et al. Probability of early pregnancy loss in women with vaginal bleeding and a singleton live fetus at ultrasound scan. J Obstet Gynaecol 2006;26(8):782–4.

[10] Hasan R, Baird DD, Herring AH, et al. Patterns and predictors of vaginal bleeding in the first trimester of pregnancy. Ann Epidemiol 2010;20(7):524–32.

[11] Hasan R, Baird DD, Herring AH, et al. Association between first-trimester vaginal bleeding and miscarriage. Obstet Gynecol 2009;114(4):860–7.

[12] Haas DM, Ramsey PS. Progestogen for preventing miscarriage. Cochrane Database Syst Rev 2013;(10):CD003511.

[13] Aleman A, Althabe F, Belizán JM, et al. Bed rest during pregnancy for preventing miscarriage. Cochrane Database Syst Rev 2005;(2):CD003576.

[14] Rumbold A, Middleton P, Crowther CA. Vitamin supplementation for preventing miscarriage. Cochrane Database Syst Rev 2005;(2):CD004073.

[15] Haas A, Maschmeyer G. Antibiotic therapy in pregnancy. Deutsche medizinische Wochenschrift (1946) 2008;133(11):511–5.

[16] Torre A, Huchon C, Bussieres L, et al. Immediate versus delayed medical treatment for first-trimester miscarriage: a randomized trial. Am J Obstet Gynaecol 2012;206(3): 215.e1.

[17] Neilson JP, Gyte GM, Hickey M, et al. Medical treatments for incomplete miscarriage. Cochrane Database Syst Rev 2017;(1):CD007223.

[18] Neilson JP, Gyte GM, Hickey M, et al. Medical treatments for incomplete miscarriage. Cochrane Database of Systematic Reviews 2013;(3):CD007223.

[19] Casikar I, Bignardi T, Riemke J, et al. Expectant management of spontaneous first-trimester miscarriage: prospective validation of the '2-week rule'. Ultrasound Obstet Gynecol 2010;35(2):223–7; https://doi.org/10.1002/uog.7486.

[20] Luise C, Jermy K, May C, et al. Outcome of expectant management of spontaneous first trimester miscarriage: observational study. BMJ 2002;324(7342):873–5.

[21] Schreiber CA, Creinin MD, Atrio J, et al. Mifepristone pretreatment for the medical management of early pregnancy loss, medical management of early pregnancy loss. N Engl J Med 2018;378(23):2161–70.

[22] Kim C, Barnard S, Neilson JP, et al. Medical treatments for incomplete miscarriage. Cochrane Database Syst Rev 2017;(1):CD007223.

[23] Early pregnancy loss. ACOG Practice Bulletin No. 200. American College of Obstetricians and Gynecologists. Obstet Gynecol 2018;132:e197–207.

[24] Blum J, Winikoff B, Gemzell-Danielsson K, et al. Treatment of incomplete abortion and miscarriage with misoprostol. Int J Gynaecol Obstet 2007;99(Suppl 2):S186–9.

[25] Sotiriadis A, Makrydimas G, Papatheodorou S, et al. Expectant, medical, or surgical management of first-trimester miscarriage: a meta-analysis. Obstet Gynecol 2005;105(5 Pt. 1): 1105–13.

[26] Zhang J, Giles JM, Barnhart K, et al. A comparison of medical management with misoprostol and surgical management for early pregnancy failure. N Engl J Med 2005;353(8): 761–9.

[27] Smith LF, Ewings PD, Quinlan C. Incidence of pregnancy after expectant, medical, or surgical management of spontaneous first trimester miscarriage: long term follow-up of miscarriage treatment (MIST) randomised controlled trial. BMJ 2009;339:b3827.

[28] Hoover KW, Tao G, Kent CK. Trends in the diagnosis and treatment of ectopic pregnancy in the United States. Obstet Gynecol 2010;115(3):495–502.

[29] Bouyer J, Coste J, Fernandez H, et al. Sites of ectopic pregnancy: a 10 year population-based study of 1800 cases. Hum Reprod 2002;17(12):3224–30.

[30] Tubal ectopic pregnancy. Practice Bulletin No. 193. American College of Obstetrics and Gynecology. Obstet Gynecol 2018;131(3):91–103.

[31] Bardos J, Hercz D, Friedenthal J, et al. A national survey on public perceptions of miscarriage. Obstet Gynecol 2015;125(6):1313–20.

[32] Surette A, Dunham S. Early pregnancy risks. In: Decherney AH, Nathan L, Laufer N, Roman AS, editors. Current diagnosis & treatment obstetrics & gynecology. 11th edition. New York: McGraw Hill; 2013. p. 7690–8184.

[33] Saraiya M, Berg CJ, Shulman H, et al. Estimates of the annual number of clinically recognized pregnancies in the United States, 1981-1991. Am J Epidemiol 1999;149(11):1025–9.

APPENDIX 1: PREGNANCY LOSS PLAN OF CARE WORKSHEET

Loss type: SAB, MAB, Ectopic, Molar
Diagnosed @ _____ weeks EGA on _____ date
Provider to follow-up with patient: _____
Initial β-hCG: _____ Initial u/s results: _____
Patient chooses (circle one): EXPECTANT/MEDICAL/SURGICAL Management
Referred to: _____
Outcome: _____
Follow-up in _____ weeks:
   Follow-up β-hCG (if indicated) _____
   Follow-up u/s (if indicated): _____
   Birth control decision (if any): _____
   Final visit completed on: _____

Abbreviations: EGA, estimated gestational age; MAB, missed abortion; SAB, spontaneous abortion; u/s, ultrasound.

Advances in Family Practice Nursing 1 (2019) 131–141

ADVANCES IN FAMILY PRACTICE NURSING

Women's Health Care for Incarcerated Women

Donna Jackson-Köhlin, CNM, MSN, CCHP

Baystate Midwifery Education Program, Baystate Health Systems, 689 Chestnut Street, Springfield, MA 01199, USA

Keywords
- Incarcerated women • Correctional system • Healthcare disparities
- Substance misuse disorder • Pregnancy while incarcerated
- Pre-release contraception • Shackling in labor

Key points
- Women in custody often have chronic unmet health care needs such as under-treated medical, psychiatric, and infectious disease and substance misuse disorders.
- Providing prenatal care in a correctional setting provides challenges because pregnancies may not be diagnosed until incarceration and release plans are often uncertain.
- Women who enter the correctional system with substance misuse require education and access to addiction treatment. Maintenance on opioid agonist therapy is not usually provided, although relapse and overdose after release is a risk.

INTRODUCTION
"Orange is the New Black," the contemporary Netflix series, may have given many a first glimpse into the world of incarcerated women, but at heart, "Orange" is entertainment. As of 2016, an estimated 2.1 million incarcerated adults [1] live lives that are far more stark than Hollywood permits. The United States contains 5% of the world population, but incarcerates 25% of the world's prisoners [2]. The number of women in custody, which includes probation, parole, pretrial, and sentenced status, continues to increase [3]. In 1980, there were 26,000 women in jails and state or Federal prisons. That

No relationships to disclose.

E-mail address: Donna.Jackson-KohlinCNM@baystatehealth.org

https://doi.org/10.1016/j.yfpn.2019.01.001
2589-420X/19/

number has increased to 213,722 in 2016 [4–6]. One reality for nearly all who work in health care today is that we will care for someone who is or has been part of the correctional system, or who is a partner, sibling, mother, or child of someone who has been incarcerated.

Health care problems for those involved in the justice system are numerous. Decreased engagement and utilization of health care lead to the need for many chronic health care problems to be initially diagnosed or addressed during incarceration. Reproductive health needs may take a lower priority in day-to-day living for many incarcerated women, whose pregnancies or sexually transmitted infections are identified once incarcerated. Recognizing and treating substance misuse disorders, mental health diagnoses, and infectious diseases are critical to address, not only for each individual but for overall public health because the systems are entwined. People in corrections, particularly those in jails, come from, and are part of a community, and will return to a community, ideally with improvements in health. However, for many facilities this is more difficult to accomplish for women than for men, for reasons that will be reviewed. A description of correctional settings, the population of women in custody today, their health care needs and issues, day to day provision of care, and special challenges in caring for women inmates are reviewed in this article.

Terminology

It may be useful to understand some definitions and terms used with regard to the correctional system. First, there is a difference between jails and prisons. Although people are "imprisoned" in both settings, they are different. Prisons are under the jurisdiction of state or Federal Bureau of Prisons or State Departments of Correctional Services and in most states, house offenders with sentences greater than 1 year [7].

In contrast, jails operate under local city or county direction. They house both offenders convicted of charges and those awaiting trial who are not granted bail, or more commonly, cannot afford bail. In most states, a jail sentence will be less than 1 year, although in some states, an inmate can remain in jail for a sentence of up to 2 and a half years. In high-profile cases, an inmate may await trial for longer than this time and remain in the jail. Jails have been called a "revolving door" because many inmates are returned to jail for violation of parole rather than new offenses. Jail stays can vary, from overnight to much lengthier durations, while awaiting trial.

Corrections encompass the branch of the criminal justice system that punishes an offender after conviction and include community-based settings such as halfway houses, electronic monitoring, home confinement, community service, and drug treatment programs that may be part of a sentence.

Probation is an alternative to incarceration, which suspends a sentence and allows someone to remain in the community under supervision. Conditions are usually mandated and violation of parole will cause the person's return to a correctional facility [8].

Parole allows early release from incarceration with community supervision. Both probation and parole can have strict requirements, including finding and maintaining employment (a challenge for many released offenders), reporting to a parole officer, not traveling outside a certain area, drug testing, or paying restitution or fines.

BACKGROUND

Women who are involved with the criminal justice system are much more likely to have the following:

- Grown up in poverty
- A diagnosis of serious mental illness
- Experience sexual assault and violence
- A lower level of education and literacy
- History of substance misuse disorders [9,10]

Most incarcerated women have had sporadic care for chronic illnesses.

High-risk lifestyles contribute to a higher incidence of infectious disease, including human immunodeficiency virus (HIV)/AIDS, hepatitis B and C, sexually transmitted infections (STIs), and tuberculosis [11,12].

Inmates are more likely to have been homeless in the year before incarceration, and having been incarcerated more than once carries a risk of homelessness after release, which is 13 times higher than that of the general public [13,14].

Between 1980 and 2016, the most recent year for which statistics are available, the number of women under correctional supervision has continued to increase. In 1980, there were 26,000 women in jails and state or Federal prisons. That number has increased to 213,722 in 2016 [15]. This increase of more than 700% has been attributed to harsher drug policy laws, enhanced law enforcement efforts, and social factors that may make reentry after incarceration difficult. More than 118,000 women were on parole, and more than 900,000 women were on probation in 2016.

- African-American women are incarcerated at a rate of 96 per 100,000
- Latina women: 67 per 100,000
- White women: 49 per 100,000 [15]

Racial disparities seen outside the correctional system are magnified within. "This is a population that is most affected by all the social ills of our country, including mental illness, substance abuse, poverty, lack of education, disintegrating communities, and broken families [16].

In 2004, an estimated 56% of women in Federal prisons, and 62% in state prisons, were mothers of minor children [16]. In 2007, 1.7 million children had a parent who was incarcerated. One in 15 African-American children, 1 in 42 Latino children, and 1 in 111 Caucasian children had a parent who was incarcerated [17]. Because there are fewer women's prisons than men's, more than half of incarcerated women have been placed in correctional facilities more than 100 miles away from home, compromising contact and visitation with families and children. Only in the last few years have some states declined to enforce aspects of the Adoption and Safe Families Act of 1997, which required states to petition for involuntary termination of parental rights for a child who was out of parental custody for 15 of the past 22 months [18]. Parental incarceration may serve as a traumatic stressor with a significant effect on the child's well-being [19,20].

Approximately 30% of women in jails, versus 5% in the general population, have serious mental illness diagnoses [21]. Dual diagnosis of mental illness and addiction is common in the incarcerated population [22]. This may suggest inadequate community treatment resources for both conditions. The comorbidities of mental illness and addiction may reflect an attempt to self-medicate, and the behaviors involved with substance abuse are risk factors for repeated interactions with the law and subsequent incarceration. Josiah Rich (2016) wrote in The Lancet that "the three largest facilities housing psychiatric patients in the United States are not hospitals but jails," and include correctional facilities in New York, Chicago, and Los Angeles [23]. Posttraumatic stress disorder is common, because many women have been victims of (or witness to) violent crimes or physical or sexual abuse [24].

ARRIVAL AT JAIL

There are no mandatory standards for health care in corrections. However, the National Commission on Correctional Health Care (NCCHC) and the American Correctional Association offer recommended standards of care, position statements, a voluntary accreditation process for facilities, and certification for staff in correctional health. The Standard Minimum Rules for the Treatment of Prisoners was adopted by the United Nations in 1957, and it specifies that medical services must be available for "treatment of sick prisoners," as well as needs related to hygiene, accommodations, clothing and bedding, food, exercise, dental care, and obstetric care, as well as care for ill infants [25]. This document was revised by the United Nations in 2015 to "reflect recent advances in correctional science and best practices" [25].The Women's Correctional Facility in which our practice provides care follows NCCHC guidelines [26].

Women enter this facility after an arrest, as a transfer from another facility, or from court, either after an initial bail hearing or after sentencing. There is a recent effort to transfer women directly from police lockup to custody, in part to identify unstable medical complications such as drug withdrawal, intoxication, or acute needs of other conditions such as diabetes or severe hypertension. On arrival to the women's facility, an initial health screening is obtained by a registered nurse. Any acute findings requiring treatment or medication should be identified at this time. Injuries sustained at the time of arrest should be assessed. Mental health status and risk of self-harm are evaluated. Urine samples for gonorrhea and chlamydia are send routinely to the state Department of Public Health for all women aged 30 years and younger, the initial screening at intake aims to identify women with the highest incidence of STIs. Screening for STIs may be performed based on identified risk factors, or by request, for women in all age groups. Women of childbearing age are given a urine pregnancy test. Emergency contraception, Plan B (levonorgestrel) and now Ella (ulipristal) is offered to anyone who meets the criteria for its use: unprotected intercourse within the past 5 days and a desire not to be pregnant. The menstrual cycle is altered by many conditions, including substance misuse, low body weight, and extreme stress. Many women lack access to contraception and learn of a new pregnancy after incarceration. Options for unplanned pregnancy include the same options and right to choose as for those who are not incarcerated. However, women may experience difficulty accessing abortion options while incarcerated [27]. Termination requires outside funding, through Planned Parenthood or other programs.

There are protocols initiated to prevent drug withdrawal complications and symptom management from alcohol, opioids, and benzodiazepines. Although the value of continuing medication-assisted treatment (MAT) during incarceration is well recognized [28,29], few correctional facilities maintain inmates on these medications, with the exception of pregnant women who were on MAT or who have been using opioids before incarceration. Risks of withdrawal from past research in the 1970s cite preterm birth, fetal distress, and stillbirth [30], although more recent research suggests that risks to the fetus during detoxification may be minimal.

A public health model guides medical care and policies used in this facility [15]. Goals of public health care include early detection and treatment of disease, prevention, health education, discharge planning using case management, and continuity of care. Linkages with local community health centers are an important part of discharge planning, and men and women are offered care in a health center near the neighborhood corresponding to their most recent zip code or address on release.

The medical providers inside the jail include physicians from the surrounding community health centers, a nurse practitioner, and a physician assistant. They provide direct care for acute and chronic problems, coordinate outside consultations with specialists, and work in collaboration with staff physicians. The sheer size of some of the medical charts speaks to the high degree of recidivism seen in this population, as well as the significant health problems that many incarcerated women face.

Common gynecologic problems encountered include the following:

- Screening for STIs. The number of women who admit to sex work, survival sex, and sexual assault in this setting corresponds to a high incidence of STIs. Pelvic inflammatory disease and subsequent sequelae including infertility or ectopic pregnancy are risks of untreated STIs. Women with substance use disorders seem needed to be reacquainted with their bodies once in recovery, because they notice secretions or sensations that we can reassure them are normal but are newly apparent and concerning to them.
- Evaluation of abnormal uterine bleeding (AUB) or other menstrual problems. Use of opioids, intravenous drug use, chronic malnutrition, and severe weight

loss contribute to anovulation [31,32]. Many women present with a history of prolonged amenorrhea while using drugs. Drug detoxification, regular meals, and reaching a normal body mass index often restore a regular menstrual cycle. Other causes of anovulation must be ruled out, and pregnancy must always be a consideration as a cause of amenorrhea. Some psychiatric medications cause an increase in prolactin levels, and many medications can cause a significant weight gain that can trigger AUB.

- Pelvic pain is a frequent complaint. Acute pelvic pain is defined as less than 3 months' duration [33]. Most pelvic pain can be attributed to a few common diagnoses, although a wide range of causes must be ruled out. Pelvic inflammatory disease, pregnancy, appendicitis, a ruptured ovarian cyst, endometriosis, or degenerating fibroids are among the most common causes. Factors complicating evaluation include a history of sexual abuse, with an estimated incidence of 15% to 25% in the general population and an association with chronic pelvic pain. Prior experience in obtaining narcotics in an emergency room sometimes colors the complaint of pelvic pain, because our national recognition of "pain as the fifth vital sign" [34] has been responsible for an expectation of narcotic medication for pain relief. Although this is becoming a less common practice, getting out of the jail and to an emergency room at any cost is sometimes an urgent goal for the woman who is experiencing symptoms of withdrawal and requires careful evaluation in order not to miss a significant diagnosis.

- Providing prerelease contraception decreases the likelihood of unplanned pregnancies in the chaotic period after release, when competing needs make accessing resources for preventative care, a lower priority than immediate needs such as housing, earning an income, and reestablishing relationships with family members [35]. Women who plan to use a community program offering Vivitrol for MAT are strongly encouraged to obtain prerelease contraception, because it is not approved for use in pregnancy. Women in the court-appointed drug and alcohol treatment program, as well as the women at the jail, are seen to discuss and initiate some form of contraception if desired.

- Cytologic screening (Pap smears) is offered using current American Society for Colposcopy and Cervical Pathology guidelines. Colposcopies are done at the hospital out-patient office. Surgical treatment is scheduled through the resident clinic. Treatment of cervical dysplasia is often interrupted by release from incarceration without follow-up, sometimes with progression and severe consequences. Education about medical care and self-care is a high priority, but situational factors preventing continued care after release must be acknowledged and addressed.

- Obstetric care is provided at the jail. Conditions that risk out of our midwifery practice, such as multiple gestation or uncontrolled diabetes in women, are seen by the obstetric residents at the hospital clinic. Many women have high-risk histories with poor pregnancy outcomes from prematurity or growth restriction. However, these have occurred within a setting of substance use, chaotic lifestyles, and lack of prenatal care. A controlled living situation, while in recovery, with careful surveillance of risk factors often leads to a healthy full-term pregnancy outcome. It is often difficult to plan for care when someone is released unexpectedly or incarcerated for a very short duration. Dating ultrasounds may be obtained early in pregnancy in case of release and a subsequent gap in care. With the exception of planning for permanent sterilization, for which consent cannot be obtained while in custody, care is unchanged by incarceration.

Pregnant women with opioid use disorder are offered opioid agonist therapy with methadone or buprenorphine. Methadone treatment during pregnancy has been in use longer but outcomes are similar for both options, with potentially shorter duration for neonatal withdrawal treatment seen with use of buprenorphine [36].

Consultations with the department of anesthesia, and with a neonatologist, are arranged. Pain management options in labor are altered by use of methadone and buprenorphine. Newborns are likely to undergo at least some degree of neonatal opioid withdrawal or abstinence syndrome. Medication-assisted withdrawal during pregnancy is not recommended, both for potential risk of preterm birth, low birth weight, and neonatal withdrawal and for the likelihood of relapse. More recent studies suggest that opioid withdrawal may have no increased risks of poor obstetric or neonatal outcomes although further research is ongoing [30].

Involvement with the Department of Social Services is mandated by use of either medication, although the positive aspect of this in terms of services available is emphasized. Many women have lost custody of other children and remain apprehensive that it will happen again. The family counselor assists in designating plans for care of the newborn. Unfortunately, fractured family structures and alienation from partners and family sometimes mean that the infant will be placed into foster care.

GIVING BIRTH WHILE INCARCERATED

Although many women are released to home or to a residential treatment program before going into labor, some will give birth while incarcerated. A family coordinator will help make preliminary plans for care of the newborn, because there is no nursery in the jail. There are fewer than a dozen facilities nationwide with nursery programs that allow the infant and mother to remain together for a designated time period. Usually one support person will receive clearance to be with the woman in labor and for an hour or so postpartum. The partner may also be incarcerated or otherwise unavailable or family members may be too far away to come on short notice for labor support. Doula programs, such as "The Prison Birth Project," which recently disbanded, have offered ongoing support during pregnancy, labor, postpartum, and beyond release.

Shackling of pregnant women has received much media attention. Nationally, women have successfully sued for injuries sustained while shackled in labor. In 2014, the Massachusetts state legislature passed a bill that limited use of restraints in pregnancy and postpartum, and banned its use during labor and birth. The bill also requires pregnancy-specific clothing, nutrition, medical care, and time for exercise [37,38]. In 2016, a survey of correctional facilities housing women showed numerous violations, in nearly every facility, of the antishackling law.

The privacy rights of inmates, which most medical providers consider a high priority, are secondary to security policies, and correctional officers are present for medical evaluations, childbirth, cesarean sections, and the postpartum period. Correctional needs and medical needs are always in a tenuous balance, and negotiating this balance can be challenging.

Almost without exception, there is no reason to discuss with hospital staff the charges that led to incarceration. It does not affect medical care and could influence the ability of the staff to provide nonjudgmental care. Safety for staff, visitors, and the inmate is assured by the presence of the correctional officer. Education for hospital staff about security guidelines, services provided in jail, and how to interact with inmates and correctional officers is ongoing.

Breastfeeding and pumping breast milk are strongly encouraged, and with return to the jail, most mothers will have visits once or twice weekly with their newborns. Contraindications to breastfeeding include HIV, bleeding nipples in a woman who is a hepatitis C carrier, and use of medications contraindicated in lactation [39]. Pumping milk in jail requires motivation, because most women need to come to the medical department every 2 to 4 hours to pump. Some women have pumped for more than 9 months. Getting a placement in a residential treatment program that includes the newborn, and sometimes other children, is a goal for many women, although there is a need for many more programs than that exist.

Women should be screened for postpartum depression, while bearing in mind that many inmates have preexisting diagnoses of depression and that separation from a newborn may cause situational depression. Women are seen for postpartum care within a week of giving birth and then as often as needed. Methadone and buprenorphine doses will be decreased gradually unless release from jail is imminent.

SUMMARY

Providing women's health care in the setting of incarceration is a rewarding, if eye-opening, aspect of practice. Having the opportunity to advocate for improving care, and providing education to colleagues, staff, and incarcerated women, has a valuable impact within the correctional system, and on our own practice, beliefs, and knowledge. Bringing students into the jail for clinical practice has been a profound learning experience. Witnessing the ripple effects of poverty, racial and gender disparities, and legislation on families involved in the system is difficult to ignore. There is a role for any provider of women's health care to become involved in correctional health, if interested. He/she should inquire about provision of care inside or outside local jails and prisons, investigate availability of doula services, offer prenatal or health education inside the walls, and advocate for women when they come into the hospital or clinical offices. Acknowledging the difficulty of having been incarcerated if it is disclosed to you and providing nonjudgmental care despite substance use relapse and recovery, or recidivism, serve to improve the engagement in medical care for women and families affected by the criminal justice system.

References

[1] Carson EA. Prisoners in 2016. 2018 Bureau of justice statistics web site. Available at: https://www.bjs.gov/index.cfm?ty=pbdetail&iid=6187. Accessed September 1, 2018.

[2] Subramanian RH, Kang-Brown C. In our own backyard: confronting growth and disparities in American jails Vera Institute for Justice website. 2015. Available at: https://www.ver-a.org/publications/in-our-own-backyard-confronting-growth-and-disparities-in-a merican-jails. Accessed September 1, 2018.

[3] Sawyer W. The gender divide: tracking women's state prison growth. In Prison Policy Initiative web site. 2018. Available at: https://www.prisonpolicy.org/reports/women/overti-me.html. Accessed September 1, 2018.

[4] National Resource Center on Justice Involved Women. Women offenders as a growing population in criminal justice. Fact sheet on justice involved women in 2016 2016. Available at: https://cjinvolvedwomen.org/wp-content/uploads/2016/06/Fact-Sheet.pdf. Accessed September 1, 2018.

[5] Zeng Z. Jail inmates in 2016 2018 In Bureau of Justice Statistics web site. Available at: https://bjs.gov/content/pub/pdf/ji16.pdf. Accessed September 1, 2018.

[6] Carson EA. Prisoners in 2016 2018 Bureau of Justice Statistics website. Available at: https://bjs.gov/content/pub/pdf/p16.pdf. Accessed September 1, 2018.

[7] Sullivan LE, editor. The SAGE glossary of the social and behavioral sciences. Thousand Oaks (CA): SAGE Reference; 2009. p. 275.

[8] What is the difference between probation and parole? Faq detail in Bureau of Justice Statistics. Available at: https://www.bjs.gov/index.cfm?ty=qa&iid=324. Accessed September 1, 2018.

[9] Wilper A, Woolhandler S, Boyd JW, et al. The health and health care of US prisoners: results of a nationwide survey. Am J Public Health 2009;99(4):666–72.

[10] Lewis C. Treating incarcerated women: gender matters. Psychiatr Clin North Am 2006;29(3):773–89.

[11] Wildeman C, Wang E. Mass incarceration, public health, and widening inequality. Lancet 2017;389(10077):1464–74.

[12] Fact sheet: incarcerated women and girls .in the sentencing project web site. 2015. Available at: https://www.sentencingproject.org/wp-content/uploads/2016/02/Incarcerated-Women-and-Girls. pdf. Accessed September 1, 2018.

[13] Duran J. Finding housing is hard but for people leaving prison and jail it's almost impossible. In: Think justice blog, vera institute for justice. 2018. Available at: https://www.vera.org/blog/finding-housing-is-hard-but-for-people-leaving-prison-and-jail-its-almo st-impossible 2018. Accessed September 1, 2018.

[14] Couloute L. Nowhere to go: homelessness among formerly incarcerated people. Prison policy initiative web site 2018. Available at: http://Prisonpolicy.org. Accessed September 1, 2018.

[15] Conklin T, Lincoln T, Wilson R. The public health burden in correctional facilities. In: Curran K, editor. A public health manual for correctional health care. Ludlow (MA): Hampden County Sheriff's Department; 2002. p. 14, 23–7, 34–49.

[16] Glaze LE, Maruschak LM. Parents in prison and their minor children. Bureau of justice statistics special Report. Washington (DC): U.S. Department of Justice; 2008. Available at: http://www.bjs.gov/content/pub/pdf/pptmc.pdf Revised March 30, 2010. Accessed September 1, 2018.

[17] Walsh A. States, help families stay together by correcting a consequence of the adoption and safe families act. Prison policy initiative. 2016. Available at: https://www.prisonpolicy.org/blog/2016/05/24/asfa/. Accessed September 1, 2018.

[18] Dumont D, Wildeman C, Lee H, et al. Incarceration, maternal hardship, and perinatal health behaviors. Matern Child Health J 2014;18(9):2179–87.

[19] Murray J, Farrington DP, Sekol I. Children's antisocial behavior, mental health, drug use and educational performance after parental incarceration: a systematic review and meta-analysis. Psychol Bull 2012;138(2):175–210.

[20] Binswanger I, Redmond N, Steiner JF, et al. Health disparities and the criminal justice system: an agenda for further research and action. J Urban Health 2011;89(1):98–107.

[21] Rich JD, Allen SA, Williams BA. The need for higher standards in correctional healthcare to improve public health. J Gen Intern Med 2015;30(4):503–7.

[22] Rich J. Speaking up for the incarcerated. Lancet 2016;388(10049):1047.

[23] Dumont D, Brockman B. Public health and the epidemic of incarceration. Annu Rev Public Health 2012;21(33):325–39.

[24] Standard minimum rules for the treatment of prisoners. In United Nations Office of the High Commissioner web site. Approved 1957. Available at: https://www.ohchr.org/EN/ProfessionalInterest/Pages/TreatmentOfPrisoners.aspx Approved July 31,1957. Accessed September 1, 2018.

[25] The United Nations standard minimum rules for the treatment of prisoners revised as The Nelson Mandela Rules United Nations Office on Drugs and Crime website. 2015. Available at: http://www.unodc.org/documents/justice-and-prison-reform/GA-RESOLUTION/E_ebook.pdf. Accessed September 1, 2018.

[26] Women's health care in correctional settings: position statement. National Commission on correctional health web site. Available at: https://www.ncchc.org/filebin/Positions/Womens_Health_Care_in_Correctional_Settings.pdf. Accessed September 1, 2018.

[27] Kasdan D. Abortion access for incarcerated women: are correctional health policies in conflict with constitutional standards? Perspect Sex Reprod Health 2009;41(1):59–62. Available at: https://www.guttmacher.org/sites/default/files/pdfs/pubs/psrh/full/4105909.pdf. Accessed September 1, 2018.

[28] Fox A, Maradiaga J, Weiss L, et al. Release from incarceration, relapse to opioid use and the potential for buprenorphine maintenance treatment: a qualitative study of the perceptions of former inmates with opioid use disorder. Addict Sci Clin Pract 2015;10(1):2.

[29] Wakeman S. Why it's inappropriate not to treat incarcerated patients with opioid agonist therapy. AMA J Ethics 2017;19(9):922–30.

[30] Bell J, Towers CV, Hennessey MD, et al. Detoxification from opiate drugs during pregnancy. Am J Obstet Gynecol 2016;215(3):374. e1—6.

[31] Fourman LT, Fazeli PK. Neuroendocrine causes of amenorrhea—an update. J Clin Endocrinol Metab 2015;100(3):812–82.

[32] Munro M, Critchley H, Broder M, et al. FIGO classification system (PALM-COEIN) for causes of abnormal uterine bleeding in nongravid women of reproductive age. Int J Gynecol Obstet 2011;113:3–13.

[33] Bhavsar Ak, Gelner EJ, Shorma T. Common questions about the evaluation of acute pelvic pain. Am Fam Physician 2016;93(1):41–8.

[34] Tompkins DA, Hobelmann J, Compton P. Providing chronic pain management in the "fifth vital sign" era: historical and treatment perspectives on a modern-day medical dilemma. Drug Alcohol Depend 2017;173(supplement 1):s11–21.

[35] Ramaswamy M, Chen H-F, Cropsey KL, et al. Highly effective birth control use before and after women's incarceration. J Womens Health 2015;24(6):530–9.

[36] Boyars L, Guille C. Treatment of perinatal opioid use disorder. Obstet Gynecol Clin North Am 2018;45(3):511–24.

[37] Breaking promises. Violations of the Massachusetts pregnancy standards and anti-shackling law. A report by the prison birth project &prisoners' legal services of Massachusetts. Available at: http://www.plsma.org/wp-content/uploads/2016/05/Breaking-Promises May2016.pdf. Accessed September 1, 2018.

[38] Massachusetts General Laws chapter 127 § 118. Pregnant and postpartum inmates; standards of care; use of restraints. Effective May 15, 2014.
[39] Breastfeeding and special circumstances: Hepatitis B or C infections Center for Disease Control and Prevention web site. Available at: https://www.cdc.gov/breastfeeding/breastfeeding-special-circumstances-maternal-or-infant-illnesses/hep.html. Accessed September 1, 2018.

Advances in Family Practice Nursing 1 (2019) 143–159

ADVANCES IN FAMILY PRACTICE NURSING

Safe Medications in Primary Care of the Pregnant Woman
Update on the New Medication Classification System

Kathleen Danhausen, MSN, MPH, CNM*,
Taneesha Reynolds, MSN, MBA, CNM[1]

Vanderbilt University School of Nursing, 3212 West End Avenue #100, Nashville TN 37203, USA

Keywords
- Pregnancy • Nausea and vomiting in pregnancy • Pregnancy discomforts
- Upper respiratory infection • Urinary tract infection

Key points

- The goal of prescribing medications in pregnancy is to maximize maternal benefit while minimizing fetal risk.
- The alphabetized medication risk scoring system (A-B-C-D-X) for medications in pregnancy and lactation is no longer being used.
- The US Food and Drug Administration medication labeling requires a summary of risks, benefits, and clinical considerations for medications taken by women who are pregnant or lactating, and by men and women with reproductive potential.
- High-quality evidence offering guidance when prescribing peripartum medications is limited; however, many medications used for primary care complaints have been safely used for many years with few adverse effects.

INTRODUCTION

Approximately 3% of infants born in United States each year will have congenital or developmental abnormalities, and 3% of these abnormalities may be caused by medication exposure [1]. Most women report prescription

Disclosure Statement: Neither author has any relationship with a commercial company that has a direct financial interest in subject matter or materials discussed in article or with a company making a competing product.

[1]Present address: 722 Holland Ridge Drive, Lavergne, TN 37086.

*Corresponding author. 3212 West End Avenue #100, Nashville, TN 37203. E-mail address: Kathleen.danhausen@gmail.com

https://doi.org/10.1016/j.yfpn.2018.12.007
2589-420X/19/

or over-the-counter medication use during the first trimester of pregnancy, when the potential for reproductive effects is greatest [2]. Clinical trials for emerging medications are rarely conducted on pregnant women owing to safety and ethical concerns; thus, most drugs come to the marketplace without fetal safety data. Most of the available data emerge from pregnancy exposure registries, case studies, and ongoing research studies that are primarily observational. Although important, such data have innate limitations because researchers are unable to control for variables that may also contribute to the presence or absence of birth defects [1,3]. Furthermore, because birth defects are rare, studies must include thousands of pregnant women to show significant differences between infants exposed and not exposed to a medication. This lack of well-controlled medication safety data makes it difficult to counsel clients making treatment decisions in pregnancy [1,3].

Primary care providers treat pregnant women seeking help managing common pregnancy-related concerns or who are experiencing illness. This article provides an overview of changes to the pregnancy safety information the US Food and Drug Administration (FDA) requires on medication labels. The remainder of this article will discuss safe medications for the treatment of 3 primary care conditions experienced in pregnancy: nausea and vomiting, upper respiratory infections (URIs), and urinary tract infections (UTIs). Many of the medications used to treat these common disorders were approved before 2001 and are not subject to the new labeling requirements. This article presents safety and other clinical considerations to assist prescribers in caring for pregnant women experiencing these conditions.

FOOD AND DRUG ADMINISTRATION REQUIREMENTS FOR MEDICATION LABELING FOR PREGNANCY, LACTATION, AND REPRODUCTIVE POTENTIAL

Medical providers caring for pregnant women are familiar with the alphabetized categories (A-B-C-D-X) used by the FDA since 1980 to rank the teratogenic risk of medications during pregnancy. Pharmaceutical companies, not the FDA, assigned medication categories. This labeling system, presented in Table 1, became problematic because it oversimplified and potentially exaggerated a medication's relative safety or risk [3]. Under this system, medication risk did not increase by category nor did medications within the same category pose the same risk. Only fetal risk was considered, with no account for the maternal risk of untreated disease. Moreover, the system did not allow for data ambiguity or differences in outcome related to dose, duration, frequency, route, or gestational timing of exposure [3]. Indeed it seems that many teratogenic drugs have a dosing threshold, below which no abnormalities have been observed [4].

In 2015, the FDA implemented the Pregnancy Lactation Labeling Rule, requiring clear descriptions of medication risk during pregnancy, birth, lactation, and while men and women are fertile [5]. These guidelines,

Table 1
Historical US Food and Drug Administration pregnancy risk categories

Risk category	Definition
A	Adequate and well-controlled studies in pregnant women indicate no fetal risk.
B	Animal studies do not demonstrate fetal risk and no adequate or well-controlled human studies are available or animal studies have shown an adverse effect that has not been replicated in well-controlled human studies.
C	Well-controlled human studies are lacking and animal studies are unavailable or indicate adverse effects to the fetus.
D	Human studies or investigational or postmarketing data indicate fetal risk; benefits may be acceptable despite potential risks.
X	Animal/human studies or investigational or postmarketing data indicate fetal risk that clearly outweighs any possible benefit.

Data from Food and Drug Administration, HHS. Content and format of labeling for human prescription drug and biological products; requirements for pregnancy and lactation labeling. Final rule. Fed Reg 2008;73:30831–68.

presented in Table 2, mandate a narrative summary of available evidence and a discussion of risks and benefits of medication use. Dosing and monitoring considerations must be provided, as well as contact information for the relevant pregnancy exposure registries. For those of childbearing age, labels should indicate when there are fertility effects associated with the drug, or if contraception or pregnancy testing is necessary for use. The new criteria will help providers and patients to complete a proper risk–benefit analysis when selecting medications and considering appropriate alternatives. This expanded discussion of the risks and benefits of medications used by peripartum women and potentially fertile individuals only applies to drugs approved after June 30, 2001 [5]. Providers will need to consult alternate sources for information on older and over-the-counter medications, because no FDA requirements currently exist for their drug information labels.

Prescribing medications to pregnant women in the primary care setting
Nausea and vomiting in pregnancy
Almost all women experience nausea or vomiting in early pregnancy [6]. By definition, symptoms begin before 9 weeks of pregnancy, peak around 8 to 12 weeks, and resolve by 20 weeks [6,7]. Nausea or vomiting that predates pregnancy or presents for the first time after 9 weeks is likely related to another condition. Similarly, nausea or vomiting that is associated with fever, headache, or significant abdominal pain requires a further workup [7,8]. Symptoms range from mild nausea without vomiting to hyperemesis gravidarum, which affects 1% of pregnant women and is associated with dehydration, ketonuria, and loss of at least 5% of prepregnancy body weight [6,8]. Dietary changes are

Table 2
Current US Food and Drug Administration labeling requirements for pregnancy, lactation, and men and women of reproductive potential

Category and Subheading	US Food and Drug Administration Labeling Requirements
Pregnancy	
Pregnancy Registry	If a pregnancy exposure registry exists for the drug, the label should provide the contact information needed to enroll in the registry or to get more information.
Fetal risk summary	Narrative description of the known or expected risk of the drug to the fetus
	Clearly state whether the drug is expected to increase the risk of adverse developmental outcomes.
	Statement on the overall background range of miscarriage and live births with major birth defects in the general population.
Clinical considerations	Descriptive information on the maternal and fetal risk of untreated disease
	Dosing adjustments for pregnancy and postpartum
	Maternal or fetal adverse reactions and how to monitor for and reduce their impact
	Drug effects on labor and birth and how to monitor for and reduce their impact
Data	Description of the data used to develop the risk summary and clinical considerations, including study design and duration, animal or human subjects, drug exposure information, key study findings and adverse effects or developmental outcomes.
Lactation	
Risk Summary	Summarize all known information about whether drug is present in breastmilk, effects of the drug on milk production and composition, effects of the drug on the child.
	Data sources used in the summary.
Clinical considerations	Strategies to minimize drug exposure, for example, dose timing in relation to feeds, or pumping and disposing breastmilk for a specific time period.
	Drug effects on the child and how to monitor for and reduce their impact.
	Dose adjustments during lactation.
Data	Description of data used to determine risk summary and clinical considerations.
Females and males of reproductive potential	
Pregnancy testing, contraception, and infertility	Required if data indicate effects of the drug on fertility, or if contraception or pregnancy testing is required before, during, or after drug treatment.

Data from Food and Drug Administration, HHS. Content and format of labeling for human prescription drug and biological products; requirements for pregnancy and lactation labeling. Final rule. Fed Regist 2014;79:72063.

a crucial component of treatment and may sufficiently relieve mild symptoms. Pharmacologic treatment is available if dietary changes are not enough. An overview of pharmacologic and nonpharmacologic interventions is presented in Box 1.

Box 1: Initial management of nausea and vomiting of pregnancy

Mild nausea and vomiting of pregnancy

  Small, frequent, bland meals to avoid empty stomach

  Protein-based snacks

  Avoid strong odors, flavors, spicy foods

  Do not swallow excess saliva

  Discontinue prenatal vitamins with iron, switch to folic acid/methylated folate supplement

  Consume ice chips/ice pops/very cold beverages

  Acupressure wristbands (SeaBands)

  Ginger root powder, extract, or capsules up to 250 mg PO 4 times/d

  Pyridoxine (vitamin B_6) 25 to 50 mg PO up to 4 times/d

If symptoms persist, add one of the following

  12.5 to 25.0 mg doxylamine with pyridoxine at bedtime; may increase to 3 to 4 tablets/d as needed

    or

  Diclegis (doxylamine succinate 10 mg/pyridoxine HCT 10 mg delayed-release tablet) 2 to 4 tablets PO daily

If symptoms persist, add one of the following: (if frequent vomiting, take 30–45 min before taking Diclegis, consider rectal administration)

  Dimenhydrinate (Dramamine) 50 to 100 mg PO every 4 to 6 h PO or PR, do not exceed 200 mg/d

  Diphenhydramine (Benadryl) 25 to 50 mg PO every 4 to 6 h PO

  Prochlorperazine (Compazine) 25 mg PR every 12 h

  Promethazine (Phenergan) 12.5 to 25 mg every 4 to 6 h PO or PR

If symptoms persist, no dehydration present, add one of the following:

  Metoclopramide (Reglan) 5 to 10 mg every 8 h PO or IM

  Chlorpromazine (Thorazine) 10 to 25 mg every 4 to 6 h PO or IM, or 50 to 100 mg every 6 to 8 h PR

  Ondansetron (Zofran) 4 to 8 mg every 6 to 8 h PO

If symptoms persist, with dehydration present, add the following:

  IV fluid rehydration

  1 ampule multivitamin or 100 mg thiamine supplement IV once daily if client has vomited greater than 3 weeks

  Dimenhydrinate (Dramamine) 50 mg IV (in 50 mg saline over 20 min) every 4 to 6 h IV

If symptoms persist, add one of the following:

  Metoclopramide (Reglan) 5 to 10 mg IV every 8 hours

  Promethazine 12.5 to 25 mg IV every 4 to 6 hours

Chlorpromazine (Thorazine) 25 to 50 mg IV every 4 to 6 hours

Prochlorperazine (Compazine) 5 to 10 mg IV every 6 to 8 hours

If symptoms persist, add the following and seek obstetric consultation

Ondansetron 8 mg IV (over 15 min) every 12 hours or 1 mg/h continuously for up to 24 hours

If symptoms persist, seek obstetric consultation

Abbreviations: IM, intramuscular; IV, intravenous; PO, per os; PR, per rectum.

Data from Committee on Practice Bulletins-Obstetrics. ACOG practice bulletin no. 189: nausea and vomiting of pregnancy. Obstet Gynecol 2018;131:e15–30; and Lassiter NT, Manns-James LE. Pregnancy. In: Brucker MC, King TL, editors. Pharmacology for women's health, 2nd edition. Burlington (MA): Jones & Bartlett Publishers; 2015. p. 1025–64.

Nonpharmacologic treatments

Dietary modifications include avoiding an empty stomach by eating small, frequent meals of bland and protein-rich foods; eating crackers before getting up in the morning; and limiting fluids with meals [8]. Women should be encouraged to eat whatever sounds tolerable, and may consider supplementing with meal replacement drinks. Maintaining adequate hydration with approximately 2 L of water or electrolyte drink is recommended, and many women tolerate ice chips, ice pops, and very cold fluids better than liquids at room temperature [8]. Women who suffer from pytalism, or excessive salivation, should not swallow their saliva [8].

Several reviews of acupuncture and acupressure for the relief of nausea or vomiting indicate that acupressure on the P6 point (3 finger-breadths above the wrist on the inner forearm, between the 2 tendons) is more effective than placebo in controlling symptoms [9]. This pressure point is used to treat motion sickness, and wristbands targeting this point are available commercially. Prenatal vitamins may exacerbate nausea, likely owing to their iron content. Ensuring adequate folate to prevent neural tube defects is the primary purpose of multivitamin supplementation in early pregnancy; thus, women may substitute a folate supplement until their symptoms resolve [7,8]. Formulations of ginger root in powder, extract, or capsules have been found more effective than placebo in reducing nausea but not vomiting [9]. Pyroxidine, or vitamin B_6, is considered first-line treatment for nausea and vomiting [9].

Pharmacologic treatment

The goal of pharmacologic treatment for nausea or vomiting is to reduce symptoms while minimizing risk to the fetus. Early intervention with medication may prevent severe symptoms, especially in women who have experienced severe nausea or vomiting in prior pregnancies [10]. First-line pharmacologic treatment combines the antihistamine doxylamine with pyroxidine [9]. These can be purchased over the counter or prescribed as the time-released formulations Diclegis or Bonjesta, which are the only FDA-approved medications for pregnancy-related nausea and vomiting. Other antihistamines have been shown effective in the treatment of mild to moderate nausea or vomiting, with no association between antihistamine exposure and birth defects [9,11,12]. First-generation antihistamines are known for their central nervous system effects, including drowsiness, dry mouth, urinary retention, and constipation [12].

Dopamine antagonists have effectively been used to treat nausea or vomiting of pregnancy [7,9]. These include metoclopramide (Reglan) and the phenothiazine drugs promethazine (Phenergan) and prochlorperazine (Compazine). Their fetal safety profile has been well-established, although the quality of evidence is low given the lack of large randomized, controlled trials [9,11]. Importantly, these medications can be given intramuscularly, intravenously, and rectally to women who cannot tolerate oral formulations [1]. A randomized, controlled trial of metoclopramide versus promethazine found both medications equally effective in the treatment of hyperemesis gravidarum; however, metoclopramide was less sedating and better tolerated [9]. Because it is a promotility agent and lowers esophageal sphincter pressure, metoclopramide may be a good choice for women who also suffer from reflux [13]. Both medications are considered second-line agents owing to maternal adverse effects of dizziness, dry mouth, dystonia, and sedation. Metoclopramide is more likely than the phenothiazines to cause extrapyramidal side effects, and has a black box warning owing to the possibility of irreversible tardive dyskinesia [1]. Metoclopramide should not be used in high cumulative doses or for longer than 12 weeks [1]. Caution should be used if metoclopramide and a phenothiazine are used together, because this combination may increase the risk of extrapyramidal side effects or neuroleptic malignant syndrome [1,9].

Ondansetron, a serotonin agonist, effectively treats most nausea and vomiting without sedation [9]. Side effects include headache, fatigue, and constipation [1]. Unfortunately, ondansetron is a third-line medication because fetal safety data are troubling. A systematic review of 8 studies of ondansetron use in pregnancy reported 2 demonstrating a small increase in fetal cardiac defects and 6 studies finding no association. However, the authors reported no increase in the rate of anomalies overall among those using ondansetron [14]. Another analysis of 2 large birth defect databases showed no increase in the rate of cardiac defects in fetuses exposed to ondansetron, but the study noted a small increase in cleft palate in 1 dataset and a small increase in kidney agenesis–dysgenesis in the other [15]. The authors could not confirm that their results were not due to chance. Although it seems that the overall risk of birth defects is low, women should be appropriately counseled and ondansetron reserved for those not effectively treated by first-line regimens.

Women suffering from severe nausea or vomiting may present with dehydration and require intravenous fluid replacement [1,7]. Although few studies have examined optimal intravenous fluids for rehydration, normal saline is currently preferred because it poses less risk than dextrose solutions (which can precipitate Wernicke's encephalopathy) or more concentrated saline solutions (which may contribute to central pontine demyelization) [8]. To prevent

Wernicke's encephalopathy, a woman who has been vomiting persistently for 3 weeks should receive thiamine (vitamin B_1) 100 mg intravenously in normal saline, and potassium supplementation if chemistry studies reveal hypokalemia [8]. Oral or intravenous steroids may be indicated in cases of intractable vomiting. These medications pose a documented fetal risk and obstetric consultation is recommended for vomiting that does not respond to initial pharmacologic interventions [7].

Upper respiratory infections
URIs are the most common reason adults seek outpatient care and receive a prescription for antibiotics [16]. URIs include the common cold, rhinosinusitis, influenza, and pharyngitis. The clinical manifestations, diagnosis, and treatment of URIs are similar in pregnant and nonpregnant patients. The majority of URIs are acute and self-limiting in nature, and do not require antibiotics [17]. Prescribing antibiotics for viral URIs has led to a rapid increase in the prevalence of drug-resistant bacteria and has become an urgent public health threat [16]. The best defense against the spread of URIs is the simple hygiene practice of good hand washing [17].

The common cold
In pregnant and nonpregnant patients, the common cold presents with some combination of nasal drainage, headache, sore throat, myalgia, cough, and sneezing [18]. Symptoms are generally mild, self-limited, and do not require or respond well to intervention [18]. However, many pregnant women with a cold will seek advice from their medical provider. Symptom relief regimens include rest, increased fluids, heated humidified air, saline gargles or sprays, and a variety of medications that are targeted to specific symptoms [18]. Combination therapies should be avoided because they may include unnecessary medications or higher doses than would otherwise be used [17].

For relief of rhinorrhea and sneezing, the anticholinergic nasal spray ipratropium bromide (Atrovent) is recommended because there is limited systemic absorption and animal studies have shown no teratogenic effects [18]. First-generation antihistamines effectively treat rhinorrhea and sneezing, and their safety profile is well-established [12]. Cough symptoms can be relieved by dextromethorphan, which seems to be safe in pregnancy. Guaifenesin has been linked to neural tube defects and inguinal hernias. Although the overall quality of evidence is low, it is recommended to avoid guaifenesin in the first trimester and limit its use overall [19].

Data on over-the-counter decongestants such as phenylephrine and pseudoephedrine are mixed. Older studies found an increase in minor congenital malformations related to phenylephrine use, but suggested that pseudoephedrine use was safe during pregnancy [20]. Recent data have shown a possible link between pseudoephedrine and gastroschisis, small intestinal atresia, and hemifacial macrosomia [19,20]. Cardiac and limb malformations have also been suggested but not confirmed [20]. Sample sizes are small and the overall quality of data is poor; however, it is reasonable to avoid these decongestants in the first trimester and minimize the dosage and duration of treatment [19]. Inhaled decongestants, such as Afrin, have not been linked with any adverse effects. However, use for longer than 3 days is associated with rebound congestion [19]. First-generation antihistamines are preferred for symptom relief and sleep promotion at night.

Acetaminophen is the primary analgesic used in pregnancy and is recommended for relief of myalgia, fever, and sore throat. The National Birth Defects Prevention Study analyzed outcomes related to 16,110 children exposed to acetaminophen and found no increased risk of developmental abnormalities [21]. Indeed, several studies have shown an association between birth defects and maternal report of febrile URI in early pregnancy and no association was found in similar women without fever [21,22]. However, recent studies have suggested a link between acetaminophen use in pregnancy and attention deficit/hyperactivity disorder, especially with prolonged use and use later in pregnancy [23]. Studies examining the links between acetaminophen and asthma, leukemia, gastroschisis, and cryptorchidism have shown mixed results [24]. Interestingly, a study of 300 pregnant women who suffered acetaminophen overdoses found no adverse effects in their infants [25]. At this time, acetaminophen remains the first-line analgesic and antipyretic in pregnancy, especially for short-term treatment. If fever is present in the first trimester, acetaminophen may offer additional fetal protection.

Rhinosinusitis
Rhinosinusitis is an acute URI that has spread into the sinus cavities. Clinical presentation may include purulent nasal discharge, pressure or toothache over the affected sinus, fever, and a cough that worsens when lying down [18]. Uncomplicated viral rhinosinusitis typically resolves in 7 to 10 days and therapy includes supportive management with the over-the-counter decongestants, analgesics, and antipyretics described elsewhere in this article [18]. When symptoms of bacterial infection are present, antibiotics should be initiated. Bacterial infection should be suspected when symptoms persist or worsen after 8 to 10 days, or high fever (>39°C) and purulent nasal discharge or facial pain is present for at least 3 consecutive days [16].

Treatment is the same for pregnant and nonpregnant adults. Penicillins are the most commonly prescribed medications in pregnancy, and have a proven safety record [26]. Augmentin and ampicillin are considered first-line treatment for rhinosinusitis. If no clinical improvement is seen in 3 days, the antibiotic should be changed [18]. Azithromycin, trimethoprim-sulfamethoxazole, and cephalosporins, although generally safe in pregnancy, should be avoided owing to their widespread antibiotic resistance [18]. Fluoroquinolones and tetracyclines should be avoided in pregnancy because of potential effects on fetal cartilage, bones, and teeth [18].

Influenza
Influenza should be suspected as the cause of URI during flu season, which typically begins in October and lasts through April. The onset of influenza is

generally abrupt, marked by fever, rhinitis, cough, sore throat, headache, myalgia, and general malaise [17]. The diagnosis of influenza should be made clinically, without waiting for diagnostic testing. Pregnant women who acquire influenza are more susceptible to severe illness, including pneumonia [17]. Considering the increased risk to pregnant women who contract influenza, and the observed safety of the inactivated influenza vaccine in pregnancy, universal vaccination of pregnant women across all gestational ages is recommended by the American College of Obstetricians and Gynecologists and the US Centers for Disease Control and Prevention [27].

Pregnant women with suspected or confirmed influenza should receive prompt empiric treatment with an appropriate antiviral medication [27]. It is reasonable to offer antiviral prophylaxis to pregnant women with significant exposure to influenza; however, early treatment is an alternative to prophylaxis [27]. The US Centers for Disease Control and Prevention recommends the use of the neuraminidase inhibitors oseltamivir (Tamiflu) or zanamivir (Relenza) [27]. Treatment with antivirals should begin within 48 hours of symptom onset and may shorten the duration of illness by approximately 1 day [17]. Early treatment can reduce the severity of symptoms, decreasing the risk of intensive care unit treatment and death when compared with a later initiation of treatment [28]. Based on limited data, the dose of antiviral therapy for treatment of influenza A and B during pregnancy is the same as in nonpregnant adults [28].

Pregnant women have not participated in clinical trials of these medications. However, no teratogenic effects have been observed in animal studies and no developmental abnormalities have been reported among infants exposed to oseltamivir or zanamivir in utero [29]. The adverse effects of oseltamivir include nausea and vomiting, and rarely hallucinations and delirium [17]. Zanamivir, an inhaled medication, is a good choice for prophylaxis in pregnant women given its limited systemic absorption and minimal adverse effects. Women with asthma or other preexisting respiratory or cardiac disease should not use zanamivir [28]. As discussed, maternal fever should be treated with acetaminophen [22].

Pharyngitis
Viral infections account for most cases of pharyngitis. Bacterial infection, usually caused by group A beta-hemolytic streptococcus, can present with tonsillar exudate, tender anterior cervical lymph nodes, fever, and lack of cough [18]. A rapid antigen detection test or culture should be performed and antibiotics prescribed if streptococcal pharyngitis is confirmed [16]. Penicillin and amoxicillin regimens lasting 10 days are the most appropriate first-line treatment for streptococcal pharyngitis [17]. First-generation cephalosporins, clindamycin (Cleocin), or azithromycin (Zithromax) are acceptable alternatives for women allergic to penicillin [18]. Acetaminophen can be used for supportive therapy.

Urinary tract infections
UTIs, including asymptomatic bacteriuria, acute cystitis, and pyelonephritis, are the most common bacterial infection experienced by pregnant women

[1]. The mechanism of entry of bacteria into the urinary tract is likely the same for pregnant and nonpregnant women, but the pathophysiologic changes in pregnancy increase the likelihood that simple bacteriuria will progress to pyelonephritis. The smooth muscle relaxation and subsequent ureteral dilation that occur during pregnancy are thought to facilitate the ascent of bacteria from the bladder to the kidney, accounting for the greater risk of more serious infections [1]. Untreated bacteriuria may also be associated with the increased risk for preterm labor, low birth weight, and perinatal mortality [1,30].

Asymptomatic bacteriuria and cystitis
Approximately 2% to 10% of pregnant women have asymptomatic bacteriuria [31]. Without treatment, as many as 30% to 40% will develop a symptomatic UTI [30]. The Infectious Disease Society of America recommends screening all pregnant women for asymptomatic bacteriuria at least once in early pregnancy [32]. This screening is usually performed at the first prenatal visit by collecting a clean-catch urine sample and sending it for a urine culture and sensitivity. If bacteriuria is diagnosed, treatment decisions should be guided by susceptibility analysis.

Acute cystitis should be suspected in pregnant women who complain of new-onset dysuria, frequency, or urgency. Treatment should be initiated empirically, with antibiotic therapy adjusted or discontinued once urine culture results are received. This approach has been shown to decrease the risk of pyelonephritis and is associated with improved pregnancy outcomes [33]. A urine culture test of cure should be conducted whenever antibiotics are used to treat UTI. For women with persistent bacteriuria or recurrent cystitis, prophylactic or suppressive antibiotics may be warranted [1]. Table 3 presents safe medications used to treat UTIs in pregnancy. All antibiotics to which the offending organism is not resistant are effective.

In the 2009 National Birth Defects Prevention Study, nitrofuran and sulfonamide antibiotics were found to be significantly associated with multiple birth defects [34]. There were limitations to this large study and other birth defect studies have not found these associations [35]. However, the American College of Obstetricians and Gynecologists recommends using alternative antibiotics when available in the first trimester [36]. Antibiotic alternatives such as penicillins, erythromycin, and cephalosporins have not been associated with an increased risk of birth defects [36]. During the second and third trimesters, sulfonamides and nitrofurantoins may be used as first-line agents for the treatment and prevention of UTIs, although they are contraindicated in all trimesters for women with glucose-6-phosphate dehydrogenase deficiency owing to the risk of maternal hemolytic anemia [36]. Nitrofurantoin has also been associated with increased neonatal jaundice when administered in the last month of pregnancy [36].

The optimal length of treatment for asymptomatic bacteriuria and cystitis in pregnancy has not been determined. A recent Cochrane review found evidence supporting the effectiveness of single-dose treatment; however, this treatment is

Table 3
Commonly used antibiotics for the treatment for asymptomatic bacteriuria and acute cystitis in pregnant women

Drug	Historic FDA medication category	Dose	Clinical considerations
Amoxicillin (Amoxil)	Category B FDA approved before 2001, new labeling guidelines do not apply to this medication	500 mg PO TID or 875 mg BID for 3–7 d	20% resistance overall, but wide geographic variation. Must have susceptibilities before prescribing a beta-lactam. Used to treat GBS infection without urine culture sensitivities. Contraindication with allergy to PCN. Adverse effects include allergies, candidal overgrowth, and pseudomembranous colitis.
Amoxicillin–clavulanic acid (Augmentin)	Category B FDA approved before 2001, new labeling guidelines do not apply to this medication	250/125 mg QID or 500/125 mg TID for 3–7 d	20% resistance overall, but wide geographic variation. Must have susceptibilities before prescribing a beta-lactam. Used to treat GBS without urine culture sensitivities. Contraindication with allergy to PCN. Adverse effects include allergies, candidal overgrowth, and pseudomembranous colitis.
Cephalexin (Keflex)	Category B FDA approved before 2001, new labeling guidelines do not apply to this medication	500 mg PO QID for 3–7 d	Cross-sensitivity if significant allergy to penicillin exists. Risk include allergies and hepatic dysfunction. Not active against enterococci.
Fosfomycin (Monurol)	Category B FDA approved before 2001, new labeling guidelines do not apply to this medication	Single 3-g oral dose	Does not reach a therapeutic dose in the kidney, so should not be used if pyelonephritis is suspected. Lower efficacy than 3 d of other agents, but resistance is rare in the United States. This medication may be an option for women with multiple allergies.

| Nitrofurantoin (Macrobid) sustained release | Category B FDA approved before 2001, new labeling guidelines do not apply to this medication | 100 mg PO BID for 7 d | Contraindicated for women with G6PD deficiency. Controversy regarding use near term to avoid hemolytic anemia in an infant with G6PD deficiency. Generally considered safe for first trimester use, though ACOG recommends using other agents first. Urinary antiseptic; concentrates in urine Ineffective for pyelonephritis. Side effects include gastrointestinal upset, peripheral neuropathy, and pneumonitis. |
| Trimethoprim–sulfamethoxazole (Bactrim DS, Septra DS) | Category D FDA approved before 2001, new labeling guidelines do not apply to this medication | 160/800 mg PO 2 times/d for 7 d | Avoid in first and third trimesters unless it is the only or best choice. Contraindication in persons with G6PD deficiency and allergy to sulfa. Folate antagonist with theoretic increased risk of neural tube defects Allergic reactions are common; serious skin reactions and blood dyscrasias may occur. |

Abbreviations: ACOG, American College of Obstetricians and Gynecologists; BID, 2 times per day; FDA, US Food and Drug Administration; G6PD, glucose-6-phosphate dehydrogenase; GBS, group B streptococcal; PCN, penicillin; PO, per os; QID, 4 times per day; TID, 3 times per day.
Data from Lassiter NT, Manns-James LE. Pregnancy. In: Brucker MC, King TL, editors. Pharmacology for women's health, 2nd edition. Burlington (MA): Jones & Bartlett Publishers; 2015. p. 1025–64; and King TL, Brucker MC, Fahey J, et al, editors. Varney's midwifery. Burlington (MA): Jones & Bartlett Learning; 2015.

associated with more treatment failures [31]. Currently, a 7-day course of antibiotics is recommended [31]. Suppressive therapy can be prescribed as a single postcoital dose or daily therapy regimen [1]. UTIs caused by group B streptococcus should be treated with an antibiotic to which the organism is sensitive, and the pregnant woman should receive intrapartum prophylaxis to prevent neonatal sepsis [1]. Table 4 summarizes antibiotics used for suppressive therapy.

Pyelonephritis

Women who develop pyelonephritis should be managed on an inpatient basis in collaboration with an obstetrician. Treatment involves intravenous antibiotic therapy with a first-generation cephalosporin. If the organism is susceptible, cephalexin (Keflex) should be prescribed for 10 to 14 days after parenteral treatment is complete (generally 24 hours after the woman has been afebrile) [1]. Cephalexin or nitrofurantoin may be used as suppressive therapy after an episode of acute pyelonephritis, because the rate of recurrence is approximately 6% to 8%. This suppressive treatment should be continued until 4 to 6 weeks postpartum [1].

Table 4
Suppressive therapy for UTI

Drug	Historic FDA medication category	Dose	Clinical considerations
Nitrofurantoin (Macrodantin)	Category B FDA approved before 2001, new labeling guidelines do not apply to this medication	50–100 mg PO at bedtime	To be used for remainder of pregnancy with monthly cultures to verify suppression of microorganism. Suggested use for 4–6 wk postpartum for pyelonephritis. Contraindicated for women with G6PD deficiency. Controversy regarding use near term to avoid hemolytic anemia in an infant with G6PD deficiency. Generally considered safe for first trimester use, though ACOG recommends using other agents first.
Cephalexin (Keflex)	Category B FDA approved before 2001, new labeling guidelines do not apply to this medication	250 mg PO once daily	To be used for remainder of pregnancy to ensure suppression of microorganism.

Abbreviations: ACOG, American College of Obstetricians and Gynecologists; FDA, US Food and Drug Administration; G6PD, glucose-6-phosphate dehydrogenase; UTI, urinary tract infection.
Data from Lassiter NT, Manns-James LE. Pregnancy. In: Brucker MC, King TL, editors. Pharmacology for women's health, 2nd edition. Burlington (MA): Jones & Bartlett Publishers; 2015. p. 1025–64; and King TL, Brucker MC, Fahey J, et al, editors. Varney's midwifery. Burlington (MA): Jones & Bartlett Learning; 2015.

Outpatient treatment of pyelonephritis is reasonable if good medical follow-up is available and the woman is generally healthy, responsible, and in the first or early second trimester of pregnancy. Women managed in an outpatient clinic should receive ceftriaxone (Rocephin) intravenously or intramuscularly every 24 hours until she is afebrile, then transition to oral medication for 10 to 14 days [1].

SUMMARY
Prescribing medications during the childbearing years can be challenging owing to the lack of robust evidence ensuring medication safety. Relatively few medications are teratogenic, and emerging research linking the dose, duration, and gestational timing of medication exposure to the type and severity of fetal anomalies will hopefully provide clinicians and mothers with additional guidance. Safe medications are available to treat URIs and UTIs in pregnancy. Mixed data around maternal and fetal adverse effects require providers to adequately counsel women treating nausea and vomiting of pregnancy with second- and third-line medications. The new FDA medication labels provide clinicians with information that can be used to counsel patients and mitigate risk. However, providers will continue to look to other sources of information to confirm drug safety, especially for over-the-counter and older prescription medications that are not governed by the new labeling criteria.

References
[1] Lassiter NT, Manns-James LE. Pregnancy. In: Brucker MC, King TL, editors. Pharmacology for women's health. 2nd edition. Burlington (MA): Jones & Bartlett; 2015. p. 1025–64.
[2] Haas DM, Marsh DJ, Dang DT, et al. Prescription and other medication use in pregnancy. Obstet Gynecol 2018;131:789–98.
[3] Public Affairs Committee of the Teratology Society. Teratology public affairs committee position paper: pregnancy labeling for prescription drugs: ten years later. Birth Defects Res A Clin Mol Teratol 2007;79:627.
[4] Koren G, Berkovitch M, Ornoy A. Dose-dependent teratology in humans: clinical implications for prevention. Pediatr Drugs 2018;20(4):331–5.
[5] Food and Drug Administration, HHS. Content and format of labeling for human prescription drug and biological products; requirements for pregnancy and lactation labeling. Final rule. Fed Reg 2014;79:72063.
[6] Einarson TR, Piwko C, Koren G. Quantifying the global rates of nausea and vomiting of pregnancy: a meta-analysis. J Popul Ther Clin Pharmacol 2013;20:e171–83.
[7] Committee on Practice Bulletins-Obstetrics. ACOG practice bulletin no. 189: nausea and vomiting of pregnancy. Obstet Gynecol 2018;131:e15–30.
[8] Castillo MJ, Phillippi JC. Hyperemesis gravidarum. J Perinatal Neonatal Nurs 2015;29: 12–22.
[9] McParlin C, O'Donnell A, Robson SC, et al. Treatments for hyperemesis gravidarum and nausea and vomiting in pregnancy: a systematic review. JAMA 2016;316:1392–401.
[10] Maltepe C, Koren G. Preemptive treatment of nausea and vomiting of pregnancy: results of a randomized controlled trial. Obstetrics Gynecol Int 2013;2013:809787.
[11] Anderka M, Mitchell AA, Louik C, et al. Medications used to treat nausea and vomiting of pregnancy and the risk of selected birth defects. Birth Defects Res A Clin Mol Teratol 2012;94:22–30.

[12] Etwel F, Faught LH, Rieder MJ, et al. The risk of adverse pregnancy outcome after first trimester exposure to h1 antihistamines: a systematic review and meta-analysis. Drug Saf 2017;40:121.

[13] Herrell HE. Nausea and vomiting of pregnancy. Am Fam Physician 2014;89:965–70.

[14] Carstairs SD. Ondansetron use in pregnancy and birth defects: a systematic review. Obstet Gynecol 2016;127:878–83.

[15] Parker SE, Van Bennekom C, Anderka M, et al. Ondansetron for treatment of nausea and vomiting of pregnancy and the risk of specific birth defects. Obstet Gynecol 2018;132: 385–94.

[16] Harris AM, Hicks LA, Qaseem A. Appropriate antibiotic use for acute respiratory tract infection in adults: advice for high-value care from the American College of Physicians and the Centers for Disease Control and Prevention. Ann Intern Med 2016;164:425–34.

[17] Graves BW. Respiratory conditions. In: Brucker MC, King TL, editors. Pharmacology for women's health. 2nd edition. Burlington (MA): Jones & Bartlett; 2015. p. 549–86.

[18] Kriebs JM. Common conditions in primary care. In: King TL, Brucker MC, Fahey J, et al, editors. Varney's midwifery. 5th edition. Burlington (MA): Jones & Bartlett; 2015. p. 219–63.

[19] Servey J, Chang J. Over-the-counter medications in pregnancy. Am Fam Physician 2014;90:548–55.

[20] Werler MM. Teratogen update: pseudoephedrine. Birth Defects Res A Clin Mol Teratol 2006;76:445–52.

[21] Waller DK, Hashmi SS, Hoyt AT, et al. Maternal report of fever from cold or flu during early pregnancy and the risk for noncardiac birth defects, national birth defects prevention study, 1997–2011. Birth Defects Res 2018;110:342–51.

[22] Feldkamp ML, Meyer RE, Krikov S, et al. Acetaminophen use in pregnancy and risk of birth defects: findings from the national birth defects prevention study. Obstet Gynecol 2010;115:109–15.

[23] Blaser JA, Michael AG. Acetaminophen in pregnancy and future risk of ADHD in offspring. Can Fam Physician 2014;60:642.

[24] Jensen MS, Rebordosa C, Thulstrup AM, et al. Maternal use of acetaminophen, ibuprofen, and acetylsalicylic acid during pregnancy and risk of cryptorchidism. Epidemiology 2010;21:779–85.

[25] Scialli AR, Ang R, Breitmeyer J, et al. A review of the literature on the effects of acetaminophen on pregnancy outcome. Reprod Toxicol 2010;30:495–507.

[26] Bookstaver PB, Bland CM, Griffin B, et al. A review of antibiotic use in pregnancy. Pharmacotherapy 2015;35:1052–62.

[27] Blanton L, Wentworth DE, Alabi N, et al. Update: influenza activity—United States and worldwide. MMWR Morb Mortal Wkly Rep 2017;66:1043.

[28] Fiore AE, Fry A, Shay D, et al. Antiviral agents for the treatment and chemoprophylaxis of influenza—recommendations of the Advisory Committee on Immunization Practices. MMWR Recomm Rep 2011;60:1–24.

[29] Gravenstein S, Johnston SL, Loeschel E, et al. Zanamivir: a review of clinical safety in individuals at high risk of developing influenza-related complications. Drug Saf 2001;24: 1113–25.

[30] Smaill FM, Vazquez JC. Antibiotics for asymptomatic bacteriuria in pregnancy. Cochrane Database Syst Rev 2015;(8):CD000490.

[31] Widmer M, Lopez I, Gülmezoglu AM. Duration of treatment for asymptomatic bacteriuria during pregnancy. Cochrane Database Syst Rev 2015;(11):CD000491.

[32] Nicolle LE, Bradley S, Colgan R, et al. Infectious Diseases Society of America guidelines for the diagnosis and treatment of asymptomatic bacteriuria in adults. Clin Infect Dis 2005;40(5):643–54.

[33] O'Dell KK. Pharmacologic management of asymptomatic bacteriuria and urinary tract infections in women. J Midwifery Womens Health 2011;56:248–65.

[34] Crider KS, Cleves MA, Reefhuis J, et al. Antibacterial medication use during pregnancy and risk of birth defects: National Birth Defects Prevention Study. Arch Pediatr Adolesc Med 2009;163:978–85.
[35] Goldberg O, Koren G, Landau D, et al. Exposure to nitrofurantoin during the first trimester of pregnancy and the risk for major malformations. J Clin Pharmacol 2013;53:991–5.
[36] American College of Obstetricians and Gynecologists Committee on Obstetric Practice. Committee opinion no. 717: sulfonamides, nitrofurantoin, and risk of birth defects. Obstet Gynecol 2017;130:e150–2.

Advances in Family Practice Nursing 1 (2019) 161–174

ADVANCES IN FAMILY PRACTICE NURSING

Updates in Family Planning Care for Primary Care Practitioners

Neena Qasba, MD, MPH[a],*, David Kattan, MD, MPH[b]

[a]Department of Obstetrics and Gynecology, University of Massachusetts Medical School-Baystate, Baystate Medical Center, 759 Chestnut Street, Springfield, MA 01199, USA; [b]Department of Obstetrics and Gynecology, University of Massachusetts Medical School-Baystate, 759 Chestnut Street, Springfield, MA 01199, USA

Keywords
- Contraception • Contraceptive care • Medical eligibility criteria • Extended use
- LARC

Key points
- Understand the rationale for extended use of long-acting reversible types of contraception beyond the US Food and Drug Administration–approved duration of use.
- Understand and apply the US Centers for Disease Control and Prevention Medical Eligibility Criteria and Selective Practice Recommendations.
- Review the availability of high-quality, free online contraception information resources for providers and patients.

INTRODUCTION

Primary care providers care for many women who need family planning services. Providing safe and effective contraceptive care is an important aspect of preventive health care.

For women with underlying medical conditions, the decision of whether and when to become pregnant presents providers with great complexity both in providing accurate preconception counseling and in selecting a contraceptive method that is safe and effective for that woman. For example, women with obesity and insulin-dependent diabetes with resultant impaired renal function and vascular disease require very careful preconception counseling. It is

Disclosure: N. Qasba is a Merck trainer for Nexplanon.

*Corresponding author. E-mail address: neena.qasbamd@baystatehealth.org

https://doi.org/10.1016/j.yfpn.2018.12.005

important for providers and patients to understand the uses and contraindications to common contraceptive methods if the time is not right to become pregnant.

This article reviews updates in the extended-use data of long-acting reversible contraception methods as well as how to use the US Centers for Disease Control and Prevention (CDC) evidence-based guidelines, called the Medical Eligibility Criteria for Contraceptive Use (MEC), to select and safely initiate contraception in women with complex medical problems.

Extended use of long-acting reversible contraception methods

Long-acting reversible contraceptive (LARC) methods are highly effective methods of pregnancy prevention, with failure rates of less than 1% per year, which is similar to male and female sterilization [1].

The copper T380A intrauterine device (IUD), sold under the name Paragard, is the longest-lasting type of reversible contraception and the most effective form of emergency contraception [2]. Its main mechanism of contraceptive action is the inhibition of sperm migration and viability [1]. The levonorgestrel (LNG) IUD comes in 3 doses: 52 mg (Mirena and Liletta), 19.5 mg (Kyleena), and 13.5 mg (Skyla) [1]. Its mechanism of contraceptive action is to increase cervical mucus viscosity to impede sperm migration [1]. The 52-mg LNG IUD is also a treatment of heavy menstrual bleeding. IUDs can be placed in the uterus by trained clinicians in the office [1]. In addition, the etonogestrel (ENG) contraceptive implant (Implanon, Nexplanon) is a subdermal implant placed in the side of a woman's arm underneath the skin [1]. Its primary mechanism of contraceptive action is to prevent ovulation [1].

The US Food and Drug Administration (FDA)–approved length of use for the devices is 3 years for the ENG-containing contraceptive arm implant (Nexplanon), 5 years for the 52-mg LNG-containing IUD (Mirena), and 5 years for the 52-mg LNG-containing IUD (Liletta) [1,3,4]. The copper IUD (Paragard) is FDA approved for up to 10 years of use [1].

Recent studies provide an evidence base on which to safely extend use of LARC devices past their FDA-approved length of use [5–7]. The process to modify and update FDA labeling is a long and costly process, which is a disincentive to its pursuit for most manufacturers. As with other medications, the FDA label does not reflect research performed after FDA approval [8]. The American College of Obstetricians and Gynecologists has also cited this research in its updated clinical guidelines regarding LARC [1]. Clinicians should use the best scientific evidence to provide evidence-based care to their patients.

This article first reviews the pregnancy rates at year 1 and cumulative pregnancy rates based on current FDA-approved duration of use (Table 1).

Etonogestrel contraceptive implant

The CHOICE project, a large prospective cohort study in the United States, showed that the ENG implant (Nexplanon) is as effective in years 4 and 5 of use as in years 1 through 3, with zero pregnancies in these 2 years [5]. These

Table 1
Pregnancy rates at year 1 and cumulative pregnancy rates based on current US Food and Drug Administration–approved duration of use

Method	Year 1 pregnancy rate per 100 women	Current FDA-approved duration of Use (y)	Cumulative pregnancy rate per 100 women during FDA-approved duration of use
ENG implant	0.05	3	0.05
LNG IUD	0.2	5	0.31
Sterilization	0.5	—	1.75 (10+ y)

Data from Trussell J. Contraceptive failure in the United States. Contraception 2004;70(2):89–96.

data are from a diverse population with an age range of 18 to 45 years (mean, 26 years) and body mass index (BMI) range of 16.6 to 53 kg/m^2. Serum ENG levels did not differ by BMI [5]. Thus, these data are generalizable to a broad range of baseline fertility and weight (Table 2). A second cohort conducted in 7 countries (Brazil, Chile, Dominican Republic, Hungary, Thailand, Turkey, Zimbabwe) followed 204 women with the ENG implant (Implanon) for use in years 4 and 5 and found zero pregnancies. Of note, fewer women in this cohort were obese (6.5%) (Table 3) [6]. Note that Nexplanon and Implanon do not differ in their medication doses or method of action. The change in brand name reflects that Nexplanon has a next-generation inserter and is more easily seen on radiography than Implanon.

An earlier analysis from the CHOICE project showed that failure rates did not differ by BMI (Table 4) [9]. Although there are limited data on ENG implant use in year 5 for women with BMI greater than or equal to 30 kg/m^2, the data presented in this study are reassuring for extended use in obese women.

Levonorgestrel intrauterine device
Also from the CHOICE project cohort, 496 women with the LNG IUD (Mirena) were followed for years 6 and 7 of use [5]. There were 2 pregnancies in these 2 years, giving a failure rate similar to that in years 1 to 5 of use (Table 5)

Table 2
Failure rate of extended use of etonogestrel implant (Nexplanon)

Mean age and range (y)	BMI ≥ 30 kg/m^2 (%)	Years of Use	Failure rate in fourth year (97.5% CI per 100 woman years) N = 143	Failure rate in fifth year (97.5% CI per 100 woman years) N = 50
26 (18–45)	51.9	5	0 (0–1.48)	0 (0–2.65)

Abbreviation: CI, confidence interval.
   Data from McNicholas C, Swor E, Wan L, et al. Prolonged use of the etonogestrel implant and levonorgestrel intrauterine device: 2 years beyond Food and Drug Administration-approved duration. Am J Obstet Gynecol 2017;216(6):586.e1–6.

Table 3
Failure rate of extended use of etonogestrel implant (Implanon)

Mean age and range (y)	BMI ≥ 30 kg/m² (%)	Years of use	Failure rate in fourth year (97.5% CI per 100 woman years) N = 311	Failure rate in fifth year (97.5% CI per 100 woman years) N = 204
28 (18–43)	6.5	5	0	0 (0.2–1.8)

Data from Ali M, Akin A, Bahamondes L, et al. Extended use up to 5 years of the etonogestrel-releasing subdermal contraceptive implant: comparison to the levonorgestrel-releasing subdermal implant. Hum Reprod 2016;31(11):2491–8.

[5]. A second study, by Rowe and colleagues [7], was a large international study. The failure rate was 0.53 pregnancies per 100 woman years (Table 6).

There is currently ongoing review of data for Liletta brand 52-mg LNG-releasing IUD for extended use beyond the current FDA labeling of 5 years [8]. The FDA has recently approved Liletta brand 52-mg LNG IUD for 5 years and the manufacturer is planning to seek FDA approval for up to 7 years of use. These data will be forthcoming in the near future [3].

Kyleena (19.5-mg LNG IUD) and Skyla (13.5-mg LNG IUD) remain effective for 5 and 3 years respectively. There are no current or future studies planned on the extended use beyond the FDA-approved duration of use.

Copper intrauterine device
The copper IUD (brand Paragard) has also been found to be effective for 2 additional years beyond the FDA labeling (Table 7) [7,10].

Summary of recommendations for extended use of long- acting reversible contraceptives
After appropriate counseling, patients with an existing device may choose to have the LARC device removed and replaced at the time of FDA-recommended product life or may keep the device in place according to the data for extended duration of use. Patients may request removal of their LARC device at any time after appropriate counseling. Extension of the duration of use decreases the frequency of insertion-related complications and can be beneficial to women for both personal convenience and financial reasons [5].

Table 4
Failure rate of extended use of etonogestrel implant (Nexplanon) by body mass index

	n	3-y Cumulative pregnancy rate	n	5-y Cumulative pregnancy rate
BMI ≤ 30 kg/m²	763	0	113	0
BMI ≥ 30 kg/m²	405	0.23	127	0

Data from Xu H, Wade J, Peipert J, et al. Contraceptive failure rates of etonogestrel subdermal implants in overweight and obese women. Obstet Gynecol 2012;120(1):21–5; and Ali M, Akin A, Bahamondes L, et al. Extended use up to 5 years of the etonogestrel-releasing subdermal contraceptive implant: comparison to the levonorgestrel-releasing subdermal implant. Hum Reprod 2016;31(11):2491–8.

Table 5
Failure rate of extended use of levonorgestrel intrauterine device

	Age (y)	Years used	Number of pregnancies in the 2 y after FDA label use	Failure rate in sixth Year (95% CI per 100 woman years) N = 347	Failure rate in seventh year (95% CI per 100 woman years) N = 160
52 mg Levonorgestrel IUD (Mirena)	18–45	7	2	0.25 (0.04–1.42)	0.43 (0.08–2.39)

Data from McNicholas C, Swor E, Wan L, et al. Prolonged use of the etonogestrel implant and levonorgestrel intrauterine device: 2 years beyond Food and Drug Administration-approved duration. Am J Obstet Gynecol 2017;216(6):586.e1-6.

1. All patients initiating a LARC device (Liletta, Mirena, Paragard, or Nexplanon) for which there are data on extended use should be counseled regarding the duration of extended use.
2. After appropriate counseling, patients with an existing device may choose to have the LARC device removed and replaced at the time of FDA-recommended product life or may keep the device in place according to the data for extended duration of use. Patients may request removal of their LARC device at any time after appropriate counseling.
3. Based on current evidence, the authors recommend the following for extended duration of use of LARC devices:
   Nexplanon contraceptive implant: 4 years
   52-mg LNG IUD (Mirena, Liletta): 6 years
   Copper IUD (Paragard): 12 years

As more evidence becomes available for extended duration of use, these guidelines should be re-visited and updated.

How to use the Centers for Disease Control and Prevention medical eligibility criteria to select and safely initiate contraception

For many medications, providers can rely on FDA labels to have evidence-based contraindications. However, this is not the case for many hormonal contraceptive methods. With the FDA's policy of class labeling to categories of

Table 6
Failure rate of extended use of levonorgestrel intrauterine device

	Age (y)	Years used	Number of pregnancies in the 2 y after FDA label use	Failure rate in sixth year (95% CI per 100 woman years) N = 1000	Failure rate in seventh year (95% CI per 100 woman years) N = 717
52 mg LNG IUD (Mirena)	16–40	7	14	0.53 (0.32–0.74)	0.53 (0.32–0.74)

Data from Rowe P, Farley T, Pergoudov A, et al. Safety and efficacy in parous women of a 52-mg levonorgestrel-medicated intrauterine device: a 7-year randomized comparative study with the TCu380A. Contraception 2016;93(6):498–506.

Table 7
Failure rate of extended use of copper intrauterine device

	Age (y)	Years used	n	Number of pregnancies in the 2 y after FDA label Use
Copper IUD	16–40	12	172	0
Copper IUD	25–35	12	228	0

Data from United Nations Development Programme. Long-term reversible contraception. Contraception 1997;56(6):341–52; and Bahamondes L, Faundes A, Sobreira-Lima B, et al. TCu 380A IUD: a reversible permanent contraceptive method in women over 35 years of age. Contraception 2005;72(5):337–41.

medications, all hormonal methods are labeled with the contraindications to estrogen, including the progestin-only methods [11,12]. However, the CDC has developed a comprehensive evidence-based guide for clinicians to safely select contraceptive methods for women with complex medical problems [13]. This guide is available online and as an app for download for iPhone and Android phones (see https://www.cdc.gov/reproductivehealth/contraception/mmwr/mec/summary.html). The CDC MEC was last updated in July 2016 after reviewing thousands of peer-reviewed medical articles. It provides structured guidance on choosing a safe contraceptive method based on the woman's medical conditions. The American Congress of Obstetricians and Gynecologists has endorsed the CDC MEC guidelines [14].

Contraceptive methods are classified into 4 categories based on their safety in specific medical conditions. The criteria for each category are shown in Fig. 1.

The CDC also released an update to the US Selected Practice Recommendations for Contraceptive Use (SPR) in July 2016 as a companion to the MEC [15]. Although the MEC assists in determining what methods are safe, the SPR focuses on how to use that method most effectively. It addresses important issues such as:

- What information or screening is needed before method initiation
- How to be reasonably certain that a woman is not pregnant to "quick start" a method (Box 1)
- How soon the woman can rely on the method to protect against pregnancy
- What routine follow-up, if any, is recommended
- How to manage common problems and side effects

A series of cases that allow application of the clinical guidelines of the MEC and the SPR are reviewed here to demonstrate their use. The most effective contraceptive options are presented first.

Key:	
1	No restriction (method can be used)
2	Advantages generally outweigh theoretical or proven risks
3	Theoretical or proven risks usually outweigh the advantages
4	Unacceptable health risk (method not to be used)

Fig. 1. CDC MEC categories. (Data from Curtis KM, Tepper NK, Jatlaoui TC, et al. U.S. Medical eligibility criteria for contraceptive use, 2016. MMWR Recomm Rep 2016;65(3):1–104.)

Box 1: How To Be Reasonably Certain That A Woman Is Not Pregnant

A health care provider can be reasonably certain that a woman is not pregnant if she has no symptoms or signs of pregnancy and meets any of the following criteria:

- Is 7 days or less after the start of normal menses
- Has not had sexual intercourse since the start of last normal menses
- Has been correctly and consistently using a reliable method of contraception
- Is 7 days or less after spontaneous or induced abortion
- Is within 4 weeks postpartum
- Is fully or nearly fully breastfeeding (exclusively breastfeeding or almost all [≥85%] feeds are breastfeeds), amenorrheic, and less than 6 months postpartum

From Curtis KM, Tepper NK, Jatlaoui TC, et al. U.S. medical eligibility criteria for contraceptive use, 2016. MMWR Recomm Rep 2016;65(3):1–104; and *Data from* Labbok MH, Perez A, Valdes V, et al. The Lactational Amenorrhea Method (LAM): a postpartum introductory family planning method with policy and program implications. Adv Contracept 1994;10(2):93–109.

Case 1

Dawn is a 33-year-old woman who has 3 children. Her youngest is 1 year old and was delivered by repeat cesarean section. She has a BMI of 38 kg/m². She does not have any other medical problems. She has used condoms, withdrawal, and combined oral contraceptives in the past but she is interested in learning about other methods.

Dawn's main issue is obesity. Go to the CDC MEC online or an app and review "Methods by Condition" and search for "Obesity" (Fig. 2).

Obesity

Intrauterine devices are category 1. The mechanisms of contraceptive action of both types of IUDs are independent of systemic hormonal levels because both copper and hormonal IUDs work locally within the uterus. Therefore, their efficacy is not affected by body weight [16]. The CHOICE project had a sample of 6000 women, of whom 35% were obese, and their findings revealed no difference in efficacy of the LNG IUD and the copper IUD when stratified by BMI [9].

Implant is category 1. A secondary analysis of the CHOICE project participants revealed a baseline BMI of 30.1 kg/m². Of these participants, 28% were overweight and 35% were classified as obese. They found no statistically significant difference in efficacy of the ENG subdermal implant by BMI [9].

Depo-medroxyprogesterone acetate (DMPA) is category 1 for BMI greater than or equal to 30 kg/m². With regard to efficacy and weight, DMPA has equal efficacy in normal-weight and obese women [17]. With regard to the contraceptive's effect on weight in obese women, among adult DMPA users, one study found similar

Condition	Sub-Condition	Cu-IUD		LNG-IUD		Implant		DMPA		POP		CHC	
		I	C	I	C	I	C	I	C	I	C	I	C
Hypertension	a) Adequately controlled hypertension	1*		1*		1*		2*		1*		3*	
	b) Elevated blood pressure levels (*properly taken measurements*)												
	i) Systolic 140-159 or diastolic 90-99	1*		1*		1*		2*		1*		3*	
	ii) Systolic ≥160 or diastolic ≥100§	1*		2*		2*		3*		2*		4*	
	c) Vascular disease	1*		2*		2*		3*		2*		4*	
Inflammatory bowel disease	(*Ulcerative colitis, Crohn's disease*)	1		1		1		2		2		2/3*	
Ischemic heart disease§	Current and history of	1		2	3	2	3	3		2	3	4	
Known thrombogenic mutations§		1*		2*		2*		2*		2*		4*	
Liver tumors	a) Benign												
	i) Focal nodular hyperplasia	1		2		2		2		2		2	
	ii) Hepatocellular adenoma§	1		3		3		3		3		4	
	b) Malignant§ (hepatoma)	1		3		3		3		3		4	
Malaria		1		1		1		1		1		1	
Multiple risk factors for atherosclerotic cardiovascular disease	(e.g., older age, smoking, diabetes, hypertension, low HDL, high LDL, or high triglyceride levels)	1		2		2*		3*		2*		3/4*	
Multiple sclerosis	a) With prolonged immobility	1		1		1		2		1		3	
	b) Without prolonged immobility	1		1		1		2		1		1	
Obesity	a) Body mass index (BMI) ≥30 kg/m²	1		1		1		1		1		2	
	b) Menarche to <18 years and BMI ≥ 30 kg/m²	1		1		1		2		1		2	

Fig. 2. CDC MEC summary chart. (*From* Curtis KM, Tepper NK, Jatlaoui TC, et al. U.S. medical eligibility criteria for contraceptive use, 2016. MMWR Recomm Rep 2016;65(3):1–104.)

gains in weight among obese subjects (1.9 kg [4.2 lb]) and nonobese subjects (2 kg [4.4 lb]) over 6 months [18].

Combined hormonal contraception is category 2 in the nonpostpartum period for obesity. Combined hormonal contraception (CHC) includes combined hormonal contraceptive pills, patch, and vaginal ring. The 2 main issues with CHC use in obese women are efficacy and venous thromboembolism (VTE) risk. The evidence is conflicting as to whether obesity affects combined contraceptive pill efficacy; however, obese women were found to be less compliant with the oral contraceptive pills and thus had higher failure rates [19]. Current studies do not differentiate between contraceptive method failure caused by nonadherence and pharmacokinetics. The failure rate of the contraceptive patch in women with the highest weight was similar to the overall rate (1.0% vs 0.83% in overall group), in which the failures clustered in the highest weight category, defined as greater than or equal to 90 kg [20]. As to the potential increase in risk of VTE, although the absolute risk of VTE remains low among obese combined contraceptive pill users, obesity more than doubles the risk of VTE compared with normal-weight women not using hormonal contraception (60 per 100,000 for class I obesity [BMI 30–34.9 kg/m²] vs 12–20 per 100,000 in normal-weight women) [21]. However, this rate still represents a much lower risk of VTE than being obese and pregnant, which is estimated at 100 to 200 per 100,000 [21].

Continuation of case 1. Dawn chooses to start the etonogestrel subdermal implant. The implant is MEC category 1 for obesity. The SPR can be used to review the timing for initiation, need for backup contraception after initiation of method, need for screening tests before initiation of method, or follow-up after initiation of method.

Applying the selected practice recommendations to initiate the implant
Timing. The implant can be inserted at any time the provider is reasonably certain that the woman is not pregnant (see Table 7) [15]. With changes in billing and reimbursement policies, many practices are now able to offer pa tients inpatient postpartum initiation of IUDs and the implant [22].

Need for backup contraception. Like other hormonal contraception methods, the implant is effective at preventing pregnancy 7 days after insertion. Women should be counseled to abstain from sex or use a backup method until 7 days after insertion [15].

Screening before or with insertion. In healthy women, no tests or examinations, such as a Pap smear or screening for sexually transmitted infections (STIs), are required before implant insertion [15].

Follow-up. No routine follow-up is required; however, women should seek medical advice if they want to discuss any side effects or problems they experience with their contraceptive method. Assessment of a woman's satisfaction with her contraceptive method and any changes in health status or initiation of new medications should be done during subsequent visits. Some women perceive weight gain after implant insertion. However, recent evidence from the CHOICE project showed that the implant is not associated with weight gain [9]. The authors recommend obtaining a baseline weight and BMI at time of insertion because this can help correlate perceived weight gain with objective data [15]. The only category 4 condition for the implant is current breast cancer. If this patient were to develop breast cancer, the implant should be removed [15].

Conclusion of case. Dawn has the implant inserted. She is reminded to attend her routine postpartum visit and well-woman examinations. She is reminded that the implant has enough hormones to prevent pregnancy for up to 4 years but it can be removed any time before that if she desires.

Case 2
Andrea is a 24-year-old who has never been pregnant. She desires to initiate a new contraceptive method. She has history of pelvic inflammatory disease (PID) as a teenager. She does not desire to become pregnant in the next year because she just got a new job. What contraceptive options are safe for her to use?

Andrea has several issues to address in selecting a safe contraceptive method. These issues include nulliparity and a history of PID (Fig. 3).

Nulliparity
    Both types of intrauterine device are category 2 and all other methods are category 1. Nulliparous women have higher levels of satisfaction and continuation rates

Parity	a) Nulliparous	2	2	1	1	1	1
	b) Parous	1	1	1	1	1	1
Past ectopic pregnancy		1	1	1	1	2	1
Pelvic inflammatory disease	a) Past						
	i) With subsequent pregnancy	1	1	1	1	1	1	1	1
	ii) Without subsequent pregnancy	2	2	2	2	1	1	1	1
	b) Current	4	2*	4	2*	1	1	1	1

Fig. 3. CDC MEC summary chart. (*From* Curtis KM, Tepper NK, Jatlaoui TC, et al. U.S. medical eligibility criteria for contraceptive use, 2016. MMWR Recomm Rep 2016;65(3):1–104.)

with IUDs compared with oral contraceptive pills [23]. There is no increased risk of PID in nulliparous IUD users, nor is IUD use associated with subsequent infertility [24,25].

History of pelvic inflammatory disease
　Both types of intrauterine device are category 1 to 2. Past PID is not a contraindication to safe IUD use. The risk of PID from insertion occurs within 3 weeks and is approximately 1.6 in 1000 [25]. It is not decreased by prophylactic antibiotics, nor by screening for gonorrhea or chlamydia before the IUD insertion appointment [26,27]. An IUD should not be placed in the setting of acute PID but an IUD does not routinely need to be removed if PID is diagnosed [13].
　Andrea would like to use the copper IUD for ongoing contraception. The SPR guidelines are applied here for her method choice.

Applying the selected practice recommendations to initiate the copper intrauterine device
Timing. The copper IUD can be inserted at any point if it is reasonably certain that the woman is not pregnant, and can be used for emergency contraception [15].

Need for backup contraception. The copper IUD is immediately effective so a woman does not need a backup contraceptive method [15].

Screening before or with insertion. Providers should perform a bimanual examination to assess the size and shape of the uterus as well as a speculum examination to assess the cervix for infection or other abnormalities before IUD insertion [15]. Providers should screen women for STIs at the time of IUD insertion only if recommended per the CDC STD screening guidelines [15]. The CDC recommends that all sexually active women less than 26 years of age receive annual gonorrhea and chlamydia screening and women 26 years of age and older should be screened if they have risk factors: new partner, more than 1 partner, or their partner has an STI [28].

Follow-up. No routine office follow-up is required, but women should be taught the warning signs of IUD expulsion [15]. When the copper IUD is used for emergency contraception, the woman should do a pregnancy test if her expected menses is delayed by 1 week or more [15].
　Andrea does well with the copper IUD insertion. She is pleased with it for ongoing contraception.

High-quality online contraception resources for patients and providers

When a patient or a health care provider would like to research a particular contraceptive method further, it is important to use resources that contain quality, accurate information. Internet sites have the advantages of being easily accessible from anywhere, but many Web sites do not provide evidence-based contraception information. However, there are 2 that are highlighted here as excellent sources of contraception information. They are both free and user friendly.

Bedsider.org

Produced by Power to Decide, the campaign to prevent unplanned pregnancy, Bedsider.org is a rich source of contraception information and teaching materials. Its content "...has been developed with the assistance of many experts and many young adults as well, who are Bedsider's main audience" [29,30]. The Web site is available in English and Spanish. Its content is presented in a fun, nonintimidating manner that is welcoming to patients and providers alike.

On the Bedsider homepage, users can access the Method Explorer, which displays photographs of all birth control methods available in the United States. When a method is selected, Web site visitors are taken to a specific method page, which contains information about the birth control's use, cost, and side effects. In addition, video testimonials offer the perspective of women and their partners who use the method. This feature of Bedsider in particular is helpful for patients to see how a birth control method affects women in real life and compliments provider contraception counseling.

Patients can also use Bedsider to find contraception providers and set reminders for birth control methods that require regular dosing, like pills, the patch, the ring, and injection. The Features section of Bedsider is presented as a blog with articles discussing a wide range of contraception and sexual health topics. Users can find answers to commonly asked sexual and birth control questions in the Questions section.

Providers can access all of these patient resources as well as establish an account as a Bedsider provider at https://providers.bedsider.org/. Available on the provider homepage is a blog-style set of contraception and sexual health articles. Providers can also list their clinical site on Bedsider if they wish to identify their location for patients interested in accessing contraception. Teaching materials, patient handouts, posters, and more in both English and Spanish can be purchased through the Order Materials link, which connects users to https://shop.powertodecide.org/.

Beyond the Pill

Practitioners will also find Beyond the Pill (https://beyondthepill.ucsf.edu/) an excellent resource for contraception information, research, training, education, and teaching materials. Beyond the Pill describes its mission as promoting "...access and equity in women's contraceptive health care. We build the research foundation to transform clinical care and women's lives worldwide."

[29] Like Bedsider.org, Beyond the Pill seeks to reduce unintended pregnancy by supporting provider and patient education. Staffed by the Bixby Center for Global Reproductive Health at the University of California, San Francisco, Beyond the Pill takes a multifaceted approach to supporting access and availability of contraception, especially LARC options.

For those interested in reviewing original research articles for the information that guides Beyond the Pill in their efforts, the Web site provides a tidy bibliography of such works in its Research and Policy section. For the full text of research articles, subscription access may be required. In the same section, policy briefs are available that translate research findings into policy recommendations for health policy and government decision makers.

Through Beyond the Pill's Training link, users can sign up for online LARC training or request on-site training at their location. Continuing education credits are available for both programs. Although the online training option is free, the on-site training cost may be discounted or waived for eligible organizations [31]. These trainings are an excellent way for contraception practitioners to become more confident in LARC provision.

Beyond the Pill supplies patient education materials and clinical tools at no charge. Through the Tools and Materials link, visitors find useful resources for both patients and providers. Through a partnership with Bedsider.org, many patient handouts are available for free download from Beyond the Pill in both English and Spanish. Providers who would rather have resources delivered to their practice site can order materials for free at https://beyondthepill.ucsf.edu/orderform.

SUMMARY

Contraceptive research continues to advance clinicians' knowledge for the benefit of their patients. Data that support the option of extending LARC device use beyond the original FDA-approved duration of use allow patients to enjoy the benefits of LARC for longer periods of time and reduce the need for removal and replacement procedures. With the MEC and the SPR, the CDC has made it straightforward and easy for clinicians to have updated evidence-based guidelines at their fingertips through its app or Web site. Bedsider.org and Beyond the Pill offer free, high-quality information for providers and patients that augments what happens in an office visit. By leveraging these resources, safe and effective contraceptive counseling and care can be provided, enabling patients to avoid pregnancy until they are medically, emotionally, and socially ready.

References

[1] American College of Obstetricians and Gynecologists. Long-acting reversible contraception: implants and intrauterine devices, 2017. ACOG Practice Bulletin number 186. Obstet Gynecol 2017;130:e251–69.
[2] American College of Obstetricians and Gynecologists. Emergency contraception, 2015. ACOG Practice Bulletin number 152. Obstet Gynecol 2015;126:e1–11.

[3] Teal S, Turok D, Jensen J, et al. Five-year efficacy and safety of Liletta ® Levonogestrel intra-uterine system. Obstet Gynecol 2018;131:66S–7S.

[4] Eisenberg DL, Schreiber CA, Turok DK, Teal SB, Westhoff CL, Creinin MD. ACCESS IUS Investigators. Three-year efficacy and safety of a new 52-mg levonorgestrel-releasing intrauterine system. Contraception 2015;92(1):10–6.

[5] McNicholas C, Swor E, Wan L, et al. Prolonged use of the etonogestrel implant and levonorgestrel intrauterine device: 2 years beyond Food and Drug Administration-approved duration. Am J Obstet Gynecol 2017;216(6):586.e1–6.

[6] Ali M, Akin A, Bahamondes L, et al. Extended use up to 5 years of the etonogestrel-releasing subdermal contraceptive implant: comparison to the levonorgestrel-releasing subdermal implant. Hum Reprod 2016;31(11):2491–8.

[7] Rowe P, Farley T, Pergoudov A, et al. Safety and efficacy in parous women of a 52-mg levonorgestrel-medicated intrauterine device: a 7-year randomized comparative study with the TCu380A. Contraception 2016;93(6):498–506.

[8] Grossman D, Ellertson C, Abuabara K, et al. Barriers to contraceptive use in product labeling and practice guidelines. Am J Public Health 2006;96(5):791–9.

[9] Xu H, Wade J, Peipert J, et al. Contraceptive failure rates of etonogestrel subdermal implants in overweight and obese women. Obstet Gynecol 2012;120(1):21–5.

[10] Bahamondes L, Faundes A, Sobreira-Lima B, et al. TCu 380A IUD: a reversible permanent contraceptive method in women over 35 years of age. Contraception 2005;72(5): 337–41.

[11] Food and Drug Administration. Labeling for prescription drugs used in man. Fed Regist 1975;40:15392–9.

[12] Food and Drug Administration. Guidance for industry and review staff: labeling for human prescription drug and biological products—determining established pharmacologic class for use in the highlights of prescribing information. 2009. Available at: http://www.fda.gov/downloads/Drugs/GuidanceComplianceRegulatoryInformation/Guidances/UCM 186607.pdf. Accessed September 29, 2015.

[13] Centers for Disease Control and Prevention. U.S. medical eligibility criteria for contraceptive use, 2016. MMRW Recomm Rep 2016;65(3):1–103.

[14] American College of Obstetricians and Gynecologists. Committee opinion no. 505: understanding and using the U.S. medical eligibility criteria for contraceptive use, 2010. Obstet Gynecol 2011;118(3):754–60.

[15] Curtis K, Jatlaoui T, Tepper N, et al. U.S. selected practice recommendations for contraceptive use, 2016. MMWR Recomm Rep 2016;65(4):1–66.

[16] Lopez L, Grimes D, Chen M, et al. Hormonal contraceptives for contraception in overweight or obese women. Cochrane Database Syst Rev 2013;(4):CD008452.

[17] Jain J, Jakimiuk A, Bode F, et al. Contraceptive efficacy and safety of DMPA-SC. Contraception 2004;70(4):269–75.

[18] Curtis K, Ravi A, Gaffield M. Progestogen-only contraceptive use in obese women. Contraception 2009;80(4):346–54.

[19] Westhoff C, Torgal A, Maveda E, et al. Ovarian suppression in normal-weight and obese women during oral contraceptive use. Obstet Gynecol 2010;116(2):275–83.

[20] Zieman M, Guillebaud J, Weisberg E, et al. Contraceptive efficacy and cycle control with the Ortho Evra/Evra transdermal system; the analysis of pooled data. Fertil Steril 2002;77(2):S13–21.

[21] Shaw K, Edelman A. Obesity and oral contraceptives: a clinician's guide. Best Pract Res Clin Endocrinol Metab 2013;27(1):55–65.

[22] American College of Obstetricians and Gynecologists. Immediate postpartum long-acting reversible contraception. Committee Opinion no. 670. Obstet Gynecol 2016;128:e32–7.

[23] Abraham M, Zhao Q, Peipert JF. Young age, nulliparity and continuation of long-acting reversible contraceptive methods. Obstet Gynecol 2015;126(4):823–9.

[24] Farley TM, Rosenberg MJ, Rowe PJ, et al. Intrauterine devices and pelvic inflammatory disease: an international perspective. Lancet 1992;339(8796):785–8.

[25] Hubacher D, Lara-Ricalde R, Taylor DJ, et al. Use of copper intrauterine devices and the risk of tubal infertility among nulligravid women. N Engl J Med 2001;345:561–7.

[26] Walsh T, Grimes D, Frezieres R, et al. Randomised controlled trial of prophylactic antibiotics before insertion of intrauterine devices. IUD Study Group. Lancet 1998;351(9108): 1005–8.

[27] Sufrin CB, Postlethwaite D, Armstrong MA, et al. *Neisseria gonorrhea* and *Chlamydia trachomatis* screening at intrauterine device insertion and pelvic inflammatory disease. Obstet Gynecol 2012;120(6):1314–21.

[28] Centers for Disease Control and Prevention. STD and HIV screening recommendations, 2014. In: Sexually transmitted diseases (STDs). Available at: http://www.cdc.gov/std/prevention/screeningreccs.htm. Accessed August 31, 2018.

[29] About Bedsider. Available at: Bedsider.org https://www.bedsider.org/about_us. Accessed August 31, 2018.

[30] About us. Available at: Beyondthepill.ucsf.edu https://beyondthepill.ucsf.edu/about-us. Accessed August 31, 2018.

[31] On-site training. Available at: Beyondthepill.ucsf.edu https://beyondthepill.ucsf.edu/site-training. Accessed August 31, 2018.

Pediatrics

Pediatrics

Advances in Family Practice Nursing 1 (2019) 175–181

ADVANCES IN FAMILY PRACTICE NURSING

The American Academy of Pediatrics Bright Futures Guidelines
An Update for Primary Care Clinicians

Imelda Reyes, DNP, MPH, RN, CPNP-PC, FNP-BC[a],*,
Jeannie Rodriguez, PhD, RN, CPNP-PC[b]

[a]Pediatrics, Emory University, Nell Hodgson Woodruff School of Nursing, 1520 Clifton Road, Suite 432, Atlanta, GA 30322, USA; [b]Pediatrics, Emory University, Nell Hodgson Woodruff School of Nursing, 1520 Clifton Road, Suite 422, Atlanta, GA 30322, USA

Keywords
- Pediatric care • Well-child • Health maintenance • Recommendations

Key points

- Childhood is a complicated time with many aspects to consider in well child checks, this article will review the components and themes of Bright Futures: Guidelines for Health Supervision of Infants, Children, and Adolescents for providers working within pediatrics or providing pediatric care.
- Bright Futures: Guidelines for Health Supervision of Infants, Children, and Adolescents was updated to the Fourth Edition and we will highlight key changes made and to review key recommendations for the different age groups.
- The Pediatric Periodicity schedule published by the American Academy of Pediatrics (AAP) will be introduced or reinforced while providing care for pediatric patients.

INTRODUCTION

Providing comprehensive and frequent health supervision to infants, children, and adolescents and their families is an essential to ensuring optimal growth and development. Varieties of health care providers (HCPs) participate in this care, including those who specialize in pediatric and family practice. The

Disclosure Statement: The authors have nothing to disclose.

*Corresponding author. E-mail address: ireyes@emory.edu

https://doi.org/10.1016/j.yfpn.2019.01.002
2589-420X/19/© 2019 Elsevier Inc. All rights reserved.

American Academy of Pediatrics (AAP) text, *Bright Futures: Guidelines for Health Supervision of Infants, Children, and Adolescents*, has long provided a national standard of care for pediatric health supervision. Additionally, the AAP routinely publishes a Periodicity Schedule, which provides guidance for routine pediatric health maintenance (https://www.aap.org/en-us/Documents/periodicity_schedule.pdf). Revisions to both Bright Futures Guidelines and the Periodicity Schedule occurred in November 2018. It is important for HCPs who care for children to stay abreast of changes in the pediatric standards of care. The purpose of this article is to (1) review the themes of a health supervision encounter according to the AAP standards of care highlighted in the Bright Futures text and (2) highlight recent revisions.

BRIGHT FUTURE THEMES AND THE HEALTH SUPERVISION ENCOUNTER

The health supervision, health maintenance, or well child examination is the cornerstone of pediatrics and includes 31 visits throughout the newborn to young adult periods, even more if the prenatal visit is included. Under the Affordable Care Act, the Health Resources and Services Administration endorsed Bright Futures as a guide for those visits [1]. Table 1 outlines the themes in Bright Futures. The book comprises 2 parts. The first half outlines the themes related to the health of the child. The second half outlines the health supervision visits for each age, starting with newborn and going through the young adult years (11–21 years). For each visit, the practitioner should review expected growth parameters, interval history, and social/family history and review of systems, including developmental survey and physical examination, with highlights by age, assessment, anticipatory guidance, and plan, including immunizations, laboratory tests, and follow-up. During each visit, it is important to discuss the issues of social determinants of health, emphasizing social factors like food insecurity, violence, and drug use.

HEALTH SUPERVISION VISITS BY AGE

The second half of the book reviews, in detail, each health supervision visit beginning with the prenatal visit. The recommendations are that a family meets a prospective HCP for the child in the third trimester of pregnancy to discuss safety, newborn expectations, and family and maternal history. The book's chapters provide new clinical content and guidance on how to implement the following updated recommendations: maternal depression screening, safe sleep, iron supplementation in breastfed infants, fluoride varnish, and dyslipidemia blood screening. There also are updates related specifically to adolescent needs, such as depression screening.

A major emphasis in the newest edition of the Bright Futures text is on social determinants of health [2]. HCPs are encouraged to ask about food insecurity, domestic violence, substance abuse, housing situations, and other issues that may affect a family's health. These issues make such an impact on the healthy development of the child and have a long-lasting impact on that child's growth

Table 1
Themes in Bright Futures text

Promoting lifelong health for families and communities	The eco-bio-developmental model of human health and disease promotes a partnership between the HCP, families, and communities to support lifelong health. Promoting strengths and minimizing risks allows for the implementation of targeted interventions throughout the life course.
Promoting family support	The health and well-being of infants, children, and adolescents depend on their parents, families, and other caregivers. Focusing on the family's growth and development along with the growth and development of the child is a central theme of Bright Futures.
Promoting health for children and youth with special health care needs	Children and youth with special health care needs share many health supervision needs in common with typically developing children. They also have unique needs related to their specific health conditions.
Promoting healthy development	Some of the most influential medical research over the past few decades illuminates the nature of the developmental origins of adult disease. For children, chronic diseases start and begin their pathologic trajectories during childhood decades before clinical manifestations create functional limitations in adults. Additionally, conditions formerly seen only in older adult populations are now affecting people at younger ages.
Promoting mental health	Promoting optimal mental health and emotional well-being is arguably a core task for developing children and adolescents. Mental health is not merely the absence of mental disorder but is composed of social, emotional, and behavioral health and wellness.
Promoting healthy weight	Maintaining a healthy weight during childhood and adolescence is critically important for children's and adolescents' overall health and well-being.
Promoting healthy nutrition	Infancy, childhood, and adolescence are periods of rapid physical growth and development. Every child/adolescent's health and development depend on good nutrition. Any disruption in appropriate nutritional intake may have lasting effects on growth potential and developmental achievement.
Promoting physical activity	Participating in physical activity is an essential component of a healthy lifestyle and ideally begins in infancy and extends throughout adulthood. Regular physical activity increases lean body mass, muscle, and bone strength and promotes physical health.

Promoting oral health	Oral health is critically important to the overall health and well-being of infants, children, and adolescents.
Promoting healthy sexual development and sexuality	Family members need to consider when the discussion around sexuality happens with their children, who should be involved in those discussions, and how much young people need to know at each age.
Promoting healthy and safe use of social media	Social media use is a topic that affects every stage of health supervision, from before birth to adulthood. Health care professionals should understand the benefits and risks involved with social media use in the families they serve.
Promoting safety and injury prevention	Ensuring a child remains safe from harm or injury during the long journey from infancy through adolescence is a task that requires the participation of parents and the many other adults who care for and help raise children.

trajectory. Getting families connected with resources, if needed, is important to get a family on solid ground to allow for the optimal health and well-being of the family unit. Social determinants of health should be screened at every well-child visit [3].

Developmental surveillance

Developmental surveillance or screening remains an important component of each health supervision visit. Following recommendations using a validated formal screening tool, providers conduct developmental surveillance at each visit, with exceptions of the 9-month, 18-month, and 30-month visits. Autism screening is completed at the 18-month and 24-month visits [4]. Every other visit has general developmental screening questions embedded in the Bright Futures forms that allow for the assessment of achieving key milestones.

Physical examination

The resources highlight the priorities for each component of the health supervision visit, specifically for the physical examination; for example, prioritized for the infant visit is the red reflex. There are differences in what the US Preventive Task Forces (USPTF) [5] and AAP recommend with regard to certain elements of the physical examination. For example, the USPTF does not recommend routine screening for scoliosis and has determined that the evidence for routine dyslipidemia screening in childhood is insufficient.

Anticipatory guidance

Anticipatory guidance is essential during health supervision visits [6]. During the visit, HCPs should discuss general health topics, such as safety and accident prevention, healthy lifestyle, parental well-being, and risk-taking behaviors. Adolescents should get special attention, and additional screening should occur without a parent or caregiver present [7]. This allows for open dialogue about sensitive issues and highlights the importance of establishing the patient-provider partnership early in the relationship.

OVERVIEW OF RECENT REVISIONS TO HEALTH SUPERVISION VISITS

To summarize the recommendations approved by the AAP, refer to the Periodicity Schedule online [8]; see Table 2 for the latest changes since 2016 [9,10].

Regarding the management and screening of obesity in children, the USPTF recommends that children be screened over the age of 6 and, if required for obesity/greater than 95th percentile for body mass index, referral for intense behavioral interventions should be initiated [11]. The AAP recommends plotting body mass index on the growth chart after the age of 2 years and counseling as needed for children identified as overweight or obese [12].

Lastly, for adolescents, screening for major depressive disorder should occur for patients who are 12 years to 18 years of age [13]. Providers should ensure that the proper mechanisms are in place so that everything from diagnosis to follow-up is available for patients and families. This is relevant given the

Table 2
Recent changes to the health supervision visits

Hearing	Additional screening recommendations regarding timing; in addition, there are more specifications regarding screening in the adolescent years.
Psychosocial and behavioral assessment	More detail, including using a family-centered approach and incorporating social determinants of health
Tobacco, alcohol, and drug use assessment	Made consistent with recommendations to use the Car, Relax, Alone, Forget, Friends, and Trouble screening questionnaire
Depression screening/maternal depression	Addition of screening starting at 12 years of age for patient and for the mother at the 1-month, 2-month, 4-month, and 6-month visits
Newborn blood	Addition of recommendations for verification of newborn screening and appropriate follow-up
Newborn bilirubin	Adding that bilirubin is checked at the newborn visit
Dyslipidemia	Now consistent with National Heart, Lung, and Blood Institute and should be checked once between 9 years to 11 years of age and 17 years to 21 years of age
Sexually transmitted infections	As recommended by the *Red Book* [15], adolescents should be screened in their adolescent years.
HIV	To be consistent with the USPTF, check once between 15 years and 18 years of age.
Oral health	A dental home should be established by 12 months and guidelines for fluoride supplementation should be reviewed.
Cervical dysplasia	No longer recommended before age 21

debilitating effects that depression can have on a child's performance at school or work and on growth and development. Nationally, 8% of adolescent youth suffer from major depressive disorder [13].

CLINICAL IMPLICATIONS AND SUMMARY

As outlined by Lin [14], the American Academy of Family Physicians highlights that there are discrepancies between the USPTF and the AAP Bright Futures and time constraints of family providers. The AAP uses evidence-based guidelines and expert opinion to guide Bright Futures recommendations whereas the USPTF bases Recommendations for Primary Care Practice on the latest evidence and systematic reviews, endorsed by the Institute of Medicine. It is up the provider to best balance the needs of the child and reimbursement models. Therefore, in conclusion, the care of a child is complicated and requires resources to provide the best ongoing management and maintenance. This summary and outline of recommendations are based on the 4th edition of Bright Futures and the AAP guidance from the Periodicity Schedule. It is important to balance the competing recommendations from the AAP and USPTF with the care of the pediatric population to ensure a holistic approach that is comprehensive and meets the child's needs.

References

[1] Fox JB, Shaw FE. Clinical preventive services coverage and the Affordable Care Act. Am J Public Health 2015;105(1):e7–10.

[2] Wyckoff AS. Bright futures: includes focus on social determinants of health. AAP News 2017.

[3] Chung EK, Siegel BS, Garg A, et al. Screening for social determinants of health among children and families living in poverty: a guide for clinicians. Curr Probl Pediatr Adolesc Health Care 2016;46(5):135–53.

[4] Vitrikas K, Savard D, Bucaj M. Developmental delay: when and how to screen. Am Fam Physician 2017;96(1):36–43.

[5] Force USPST. Recommendations for primary care practice 2017. Available at: https://www.uspreventiveservicestaskforce.org/Page/Name/recommendations. Accessed October 12, 2018.

[6] Riley M, Locke AB, Skye EP. Health maintenance in school-aged children: Part II. Counseling recommendations. Am Fam Physician 2011;83(6):689–94.

[7] Irwin CE. Time alone for adolescents with their providers during clinical encounters: it is not that simple! J Adolesc Health 2018;63(3):265–6.

[8] Pediatrics AAo. Recommendations for preventive pediatric health care 2017. Available at: https://www.aap.org/en-us/Documents/periodicity_schedule.pdf. Accessed October 12, 2018.

[9] Committee on Practice and Ambulatory Medicine, Bright Futures Periodicity Schedule Workgroup. 2017 recommendations for preventive pediatric health care. Pediatrics 2017;139 [pii:e20170254].

[10] Lambert M. AAP updates recommendations for routine preventive pediatric health care. Am Fam Physician 2016;94(4):324.

[11] Grossman DC, Bibbins-Domingo K, Curry SJ, et al. Screening for obesity in children and adolescents: US Preventive Services Task Force recommendation statement. JAMA 2017;317(23):2417–26.

[12] Krebs NF, Himes JH, Jacobson D, et al. Assessment of child and adolescent overweight and obesity. Pediatrics 2007;120(Supplement 4):S193–228.

[13] Siu AL. Screening for depression in children and adolescents: US Preventive Services Task Force recommendation statement. Ann Intern Med 2016;164(5):360–6.

[14] Lin KW. What to do at well-child visits: the AAFP's perspective. Am Fam Physician 2015;91(6):362–4.

[15] Kimberlin DW, Brady MT, Jackson MA, et al, editors. Red Book 2018: report of the Committee on Infectious Diseases. Itasca (IL): American Academy of Pediatrics; 2018.

Advances in Family Practice Nursing 1 (2019) 183–199

ADVANCES IN FAMILY PRACTICE NURSING

ELSEVIER
MOSBY

Closing the Gap

Addressing Adversity and Promoting Early Childhood Development

Ashley Darcy Mahoney, PhD, NNP-BC[a],*,
Danielle G. Dooley, MD, MPhil[b], Nicole V. Davis, MSN, FNP[c],
Michelle Stephens, PhD, MSN, PNP[d], Olanrewaju O. Falusi, MD[b]

[a]George Washington University School of Nursing, Mednax–South Dade Neonatology, 1919 Pennsylvania Avenue Northwest, Washington, DC 20006, USA; [b]Child Health Advocacy Institute, Children's National Health System, 2233 Wisconsin Avenue Northwest, Suite 317, Washington, DC 20007, USA; [c]Unity Health Care, 3020 14th Street Northwest, Washington, DC 20009, USA; [d]University of California San Francisco School of Nursing, 2 Koret Way, San Francisco, CA 94143, USA

Keywords
• Early childhood • Poverty • Brain development • Early childhood education
• Toxic stress • Adversity

Key points

• Early childhood is a critical period of brain development, and access to literacy-rich environments, caring adults, and quality early childhood education play important roles.

• Family nurse practitioners play an important role in guiding families through early childhood.

• Family nurse practitioners, through clinical practice and connections to community resources, can help buffer the negative effects of poverty and toxic stress.

• Family nurse practitioners can promote a family-centered approach in order to develop interventions to promote early childhood development that are strengths-based and culturally sensitive.

Disclosure Statement: The authors have no financial or commercial conflicts to disclose.

*Corresponding author. George Washington University School of Nursing, 1919 Pennsylvania Ave. NW, Suite 500, Washington, DC 20006, USA. E-mail address: adarcymahoney@gwu.edu

https://doi.org/10.1016/j.yfpn.2019.01.003
2589-420X/19/© 2019 Elsevier Inc. All rights reserved.

INTRODUCTION

The term "early childhood" has traditionally been defined by governmental organizations such as Healthy People, the World Health Organization, and the United Nations Children's Fund as a time period from birth to 8 years. The state of the science has found that time period to be too broad, and pediatric health care organizations are currently defining "early childhood" as a time between birth to 3 years. This is an important distinction because neuroplasticity occurs rapidly and expansively during the first 3 years. Neurons form new connections at a rate of more than one million per second and comprise about 80% of all brain development during the early childhood period, which in turn means this time period is important for foundational brain structures and setting the stage for brain connectivity [1,2]. This article aims to offer guidance and support for the role of FNP in caring for those in the early childhood period and emerging science of early childhood adversity.

Early childhood is a time when early life experience quite literally gets "under the skin" and affects physical and mental health [3]. The concepts of individual differences (each individual can have a unique response to the same experience) and vulnerability genes (genetic code passed on to the child that specifically affects physiologic development) are important to keep in mind because they significantly contribute to how experiences shape one's environment and development. If conditions are chronically aversive or stress becomes prolonged or excessive during early childhood, it affects short- and long-term learning, behavior, and health outcomes [4,5].

This sensitive period of early childhood is when care and interventions are the most effective and can determine the lifelong health and wellness of the individual. Family nurse practitioners (FNPs) who care for children from birth to 3 years of age have the ability to make a significant impact because these children typically are seen by their primary care provider more during the early childhood period than they are seen in the remainder of their lifetimes. The FNP curriculum has a population life span focus, and given the clinical hours required, there often are limited clinical pediatric training opportunities. Further, it is recognized that FNPs who care for children from 0 to 3 years old often work in high need, low resourced areas, and have this patient population as part of the wider age range patient pool.

The importance of FNPs caring for young children should not be overlooked. There is limited literature that addresses FNPs caring for pediatric patients, and scant articles specifically addressing care of children from birth to 3 years of age. In 2010, a survey of a random national sample of 1000 FNPs with a response rate of 75.9% showed 66% of FNPs provide care to children and 54% of them reported that children represented less than 25% of their patient population [6]. There is evidence for FNPs supporting breastfeeding [7], pediatric clinical guidelines [8–10], and pediatric culturally competent care [11]. None of the articles that were found specifically addressed this critical period in early development and the role the FNP brings in offering astute assessment of these patients as well as anticipatory guidance to families.

Resources not specific to the FNP but critical to those delivering primary care to children from birth to 3 years of age are the Bright Futures Pocket Guide, the Healthy Steps program, HealthyChildren.org, National Resource Center for Patient/Family Centered Medical Home, and Education in Quality Improvement for Pediatric Practice. These guides focus on the 2 most important parts of an early childhood primary care visit: evaluating developmental milestones and planning for anticipatory guidance [12]. Nevertheless, these might not elucidate the importance of recognizing adversity and promoting trauma-informed care and early home environments. A caring adult who is consistently present can positively ameliorate certain types of stress. Achieving developmental milestones and breakthrough outcomes for young children facing adversity requires supporting the adults who care for them [13].

This paper strives to highlight aspects of the early childhood primary care visit that are critical for the FNP to promote optimal early brain and child development. Healthy brain development requires enrichment from early language and caregiver engagement; protection from adverse childhood experiences (ACEs), especially in impoverished settings that can lead to toxic stress; and safe, stable, and nurturing relationships.

POVERTY AS A SOCIAL DETERMINANT OF HEALTH

Social determinants of health (SDH or SDOH) are defined by the Centers for Disease Control and Prevention as "conditions in the environments in which people are born, live, learn, work, play, worship, and age that affect a wide range of health, functioning, and quality-of-life outcomes and risks" [14,15]. An in-depth analysis of each SDOH is beyond the scope of this article, but given the high rates of childhood poverty, the authors focus on the effect of economic stability on early childhood health and development.

Poverty is defined by the US government based on income and family size, and the threshold is adjusted annually based on inflation. Poverty exists in every community—urban, suburban, and rural—and children are the poorest members of our society. In 2016, approximately 13% of the US population lived in poverty, including 18% of US children (more than 13 million children) [16]. Although poverty rates declined between 2014 and 2016 across all demographics, disparities remain. Black, Hispanic, and American Indian/Alaska Native children are 3 times more likely to live in poverty than are white and Asian children. Among immigrants, naturalized citizens have the lowest poverty rates, followed by US-born citizens; noncitizens are at highest risk of living in poverty [16].

Children born into poverty, and who persistently live in poor conditions, are at risk for several health and developmental challenges throughout their lives. Poverty has negative effects on birthweight, infant mortality, immunization rates, nutrition, language, and social development. Children living in poverty are also more likely to be exposed to violence and suffer from injury and chronic illnesses [17]. Moreover, the effects of persistent poverty can lead to toxic stress and can alter the way a young child's brain develops, which can lead to lower educational attainment and higher rates of crime, teen pregnancy, and substance abuse.

Federal antipoverty programs aim not only to provide economic stability to individuals and families but also to mitigate these long-term effects of poverty. Several programs specifically are designed to support early childhood development, including those that provide access to health care through Medicaid and the Child Health Insurance Program (CHIP), early education (such as Head Start and Early Head Start), quality child care, as well as affordable housing and home visiting. Perhaps the most widely used programs are those providing critical nutrition assistance, such as the Women, Infants, and Children Program (WIC); Supplemental Nutrition Assistance Program (SNAP, formerly the "food stamps" program); school meals; and summer feeding programs. Without these resources, it is estimated that nearly 1 in 3 children would live in poverty instead of 1 in 5 [17].

ADVERSE CHILDHOOD EXPERIENCES

The groundbreaking 1998 study on ACEs has greatly expanded scientific and public health understanding of the relationship between early adversity and later adult health. In this study of more than 17,000 adults, two-thirds reported having at least one ACE, defined as having experienced one of the following before 18 years of age:

Abuse: psychological, physical, or sexual.

Neglect: emotional or physical.

Household dysfunction: exposure in the home to substance abuse, mental illness or suicide attempt, parental separation or divorce, incarceration, or violence to the mother.

ACEs clustered, with nearly 90% of those who reported one ACE reporting at least one additional ACE. One in eight participants reported 4 or more ACEs [18]. Strikingly, the researchers noted a dose-response relationship between early adversity and adult behaviors and illness, with a greater number of ACEs leading to poorer health in adulthood. Individuals who reported 4 or more ACEs had a 4- to 12-fold increased risk for alcohol and drug abuse, depression, and suicide attempts and at least a 2-fold increased risk of smoking and risky sexual behavior. These individuals were also much more likely to develop cancer, heart disease, chronic lung disease, liver disease, and other physical illnesses, even if they did not have risk behaviors such as smoking and substance abuse. Notably, the study population was largely educated, white, and all had health insurance through Kaiser Permanente. In short, the accumulation of adversities in childhood has deleterious effects on long-term behaviors and health, regardless of one's socioeconomic status.

FNPs should be aware of how ACEs currently manifest. Since the publication of the original ACEs study, the list of ACEs has been expanded to include neighborhood violence, racial/ethnic discrimination, economic hardship, and other factors [19]. Economic hardship and parental divorce or separation are the most common ACEs reported nationally and in all states. Nearly half of all children in the United States have experienced at least one ACE, and 1 in 10 children has experienced 3 or more ACEs, placing them at high risk for chronic illness in adulthood. Young children exposed to 5 or more significant adverse experiences in the first 3 years of childhood face a 76% likelihood of having one or more delays in their language, emotional, or brain development [20]. Disparities in race occur, with 61% of black non-Hispanic children and 51% of Hispanic children having experienced at least one ACE, compared with 40% of white non-Hispanic children and 23% of Asian non-Hispanic children [21].

Exactly how ACEs affect long-term health is still not fully clear, but research suggests that early adversity causes an overdose of stress hormones. In the absence of a supporting and stable environment, this can lead to a toxic stress response involving chemical and structural changes to a child's brain, blood vessels, lymph nodes, and adrenal glands and can change how one's DNA is expressed. This can decrease the body's ability to physiologically protect itself from damage and thereby increase the risk of adult illnesses, particularly those caused by chronic inflammation [22]. In the pediatric setting, the adult illnesses may not yet be evident, but children experiencing toxic stress may present with problems with bladder and bowel control, sleeping, eating, learning and concentrating, as well as symptoms of depression, anxiety, and posttraumatic stress.

ADDRESSING ADVERSE CHILDHOOD EXPERIENCES AND POVERTY

Although ACEs and poverty may not be wholly preventable, clinicians who care for children are in a unique position to help families mitigate the negative effects of these experiences, thereby changing the trajectory of a child's life. The first step in recognizing these issues in the clinical setting is to screen families, which can take various forms. There is a growing body of literature in support of screening for ACEs, but as of this writing, there are no validated screening tools for ACEs and no universal guidelines for screening. FNPs should become familiar with various screeners that assess for stress and trauma broadly and for ACEs specifically; a summary of tools is available on the American Academy of Pediatrics (AAP) Website [23]. Universal screening questions have also been suggested as an alternative to more formal screening tools, such as asking a parent, "Since the last time I saw your child, has anything really scary or upsetting happened to your child or anyone in your family?" [24]. The FNP's response to a positive screen may range from reassurance, to referral to a mental health provider, to connecting to resilience-building parenting programs.

The 2016 AAP policy statement on poverty and child health recommends pediatricians screen families for basic needs such as food, housing, and heat and connect them with community-based resources and programs (such as WIC, SNAP, and others that were previously mentioned) that address those needs. As with ACEs screening, there are several available tools to screen for the effects of poverty [17,25,26]. The AAP recommends screening for food insecurity using a validated "Hunger Vital Sign" 2-question screener (Table 1) [27,28]. The question, "Do you have difficulty making ends meet at the end of the month?" has 98% specificity for identifying families who may need to be connected to resources [25]. The decision to screen for ACEs and poverty, including which questions or tools to use, depends on a practice's workflows and staffing, availability of resources within the practice and in the community, and incentives such as insurance reimbursement.

Animal and human studies show that positive care giving and nurturing in the early years can help buffer responses to stress, boost immunity, and reduce the risk of adverse adult behaviors and illness [29–31]. The role of the FNP is to take a family-centered approach that can build resilience in the child, family, and community [22,32]. This can include providing routine anticipatory guidance to build parents' understanding of normal child development and to identify support systems for the family; incorporating evidence-based programs such as Reach Out and Read that promote child development and child-parent bonding [33,34]; and connecting families to community resources that build stress-buffering capacity, such as nurse home visiting programs, and positive parenting programs such as Triple P [22,35].

EARLY CHILDHOOD EDUCATION: A CRITICAL INGREDIENT FOR DEVELOPMENT

Brain development can be influenced by positive factors, such as high-quality early childhood educational experiences [36]. Early Childhood Education (ECE) improves academic outcomes; children who attend ECE have lower rates of grade retention and placement in special education, as well as improved math and reading scores and school readiness [37,38]. Enrollment in ECE improves economic outcomes for children.

Families choose a child care option based on multiple factors, including schedule, convenience, curriculum, and affordability, so the decision needs to be tailored to the needs of each individual family. This section focuses on the benefits of early childhood education, the impact of ECE on life course outcomes, and the health issues commonly encountered in ECE settings. Young children are cared for in a variety of settings as they grow, and parents

Table 1			
US department of agriculture screening tool for risk of food insecurity			
	Often true	Sometimes true	Never true
1. "Within the past 12 mo we worried whether our food would run out before we got money to buy more."			
2. "Within the past 12 mo the food we bought just didn't last and we didn't have money to get more."			

Data from Hager ER, Quigg AM, Black MM, et al. Development and validity of a 2-item screen to identify families at risk for food insecurity. Pediatrics 2010;126(1):26.

often consult child health providers about the optimal setting for their child [39,40]. Many parents use informal "day-care" arrangements that are not subject to licensing and regulation, where child care is provided by a parent, relative, or nonrelative such as a nanny, neighbor, or friend, takes place in the child's home or the provider's home, and may not have an educational curriculum [41]. Early childhood education centers, which include Early Head Start programs, Head Start programs, community drop-in centers, and nursery and pre-kindergarten programs in school settings, are licensed and regulated, with requirements that depend on the state in which they are located. The AAP offers guidance on how child health providers can help families identify and select high-quality early child care options [42]. Quality ECE has a significant return on investment. Examples include the High/Scope Perry Preschool Program and Carolina Abecedarian Project, which have demonstrated higher earnings, lower rates of incarceration, improved adult health outcomes, and a reduction in academic achievement gaps among adults enrolled in ECE programs as young children [43–45].

FNPs should recognize the common health issues that arise in ECE settings, including ear infections, upper respiratory infections, gastrointestinal illnesses, and behavioral issues, as well as be familiar with policies that allow children to return to ECE after an illness [46]. Providers can communicate and coordinate with ECE personnel or school nurses, when available, to optimize the care of children across settings. In the transition to preschool years, providers can serve as an important link to behavioral health services for students and families and help mitigate the risk of suspension and expulsions in ECE settings. Preschool children are 3 times more likely to be expelled than children in grades K–12 [47].

Further, it is important for FNPs to know that there are racial disparities in the application of school discipline, linked to implicit bias on the part of ECE staff, with black children representing a disproportionate number of children who are suspended in preschool [48,49]. Given the strong correlation between health and educational attainment [43–45], health care providers play a key role in addressing these racial disparities, which includes taking evidence-based assessments to evaluate one's own implicit biases such as the online Race Implicit Association Test [50] and contacting a child's teacher or school administrators to discuss health and educational support needed to ensure the child's academic success.

HIGH-QUALITY LANGUAGE INTERACTIONS AND HEALTH

Within the medical home that the FNP is providing, the foundational element surrounding anticipatory guidance for parent-/caregiver–child interaction often begins with language. Language is an incredibly powerful precursor to literacy and anticipatory guidance, discussion, and emphasis should be woven into well-child visits with families to optimize early learning and literacy. Rich early language exposure delivered by caregivers in the context of engaged adult–infant interaction provides the foundation for children's future educational achievement and health. Thus, talking to children in both their native and secondary languages in higher volumes must start early with their first and best teachers, their parents and caregivers. Language and cognitive development depends on early language exposure provided by parents or caregivers. Evidence suggests that the number of words spoken to a child in the first 3 years of life strongly predicts both concurrent and future language skills and cognitive functioning [51–58]. In addition to the quantity of words, research suggests that the quality of language input is essential for advancing language learning. The rich, back-and-forth interaction between parent and child that supports the child's brain and language development has been termed "language nutrition" [59].

The trajectory of a child's life can be dramatically changed if parents are educated to understand the importance of language, are coached to provide language nutrition to their baby, and build the habit of talking to their infant. This is key anticipatory guidance for FNPs to provide to families of young children. Research has identified the early language and preliteracy skills are necessary to support infants, toddlers, and young children in learning to read. FNPs can help guide families to translate this knowledge into improved education and health outcomes (Fig. 1). There are a host of programs, not limited to: Reach Out and Read, Talking is Teaching, Vroom, Thirty Million Words, Hablame Bebe (Fig. 2), and others (Table 2). According to the 2017 Nation's Report Card by the National Assessment of Educational Progress, just 37% of the nation's fourth graders scored at the proficient level or above in reading [60]. Data from the landmark Hart and Risley "word-gap" study affirm that building strong language is foundational for learning in every

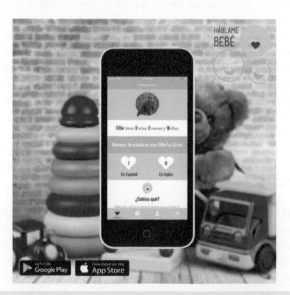

Fig. 1. "Háblame Bebé" is an app to help Hispanic families reduce the Word Gap and promote bilingualism. (*Courtesy of* Melissa Baralt, PhD, Miami, Florida.)

℞ FOR LANGUAGE — Name: ____ Date: ____ Next Appt: ____

GEORGIA WIC — TALK WITH ME BABY

Talk

- [ ] When feeding your baby, use that time to tell them a story about something happy you remember from your childhood.
- [ ] While preparing a meal, sit your baby safely in their highchair and talk about what you are cooking.
- [ ] At mealtime, say the names of foods out loud as your baby eats.
- [ ] ____

Play

- [ ] Play with your food! Spread bite-sized pieces of food on the table to create shapes and pictures. Talk about it with your baby.
- [ ] Show your baby different colored fruits and vegetables and let them interact with what interests them.
- [ ] Turn on music and hold your baby as you gently dance around.
- [ ] ____

Read

- [ ] Get a picture book and let your baby lead as you narrate what they are looking at.
- [ ] Identify food at the grocery store out loud, and read packages and signs to your baby.
- [ ] When out for a walk, point out and read street signs to your baby.
- [ ] ____

Sing

- [ ] Sing your baby a song by spelling out the letters of your favorite healthy foods.
- [ ] While you prepare dinner, make up a song about what you are cooking.
- [ ] Sing to ask your baby what they would like to eat, and give them time to respond.
- [ ] ____

LEARN MORE ABOUT LANGUAGE NUTRITION AND HOW TO TALK WITH YOUR BABY BY VISITING TALKWITHMEBABY.ORG

Fig. 2. Talk with Me Baby prescription pads offered by Georgia WIC. (*From* Technological Solutions for Provider and Caregiver Language Nutrition Training, Talk with Me Baby. Available at: http://www.talkwithmebaby.org/training_resources.)

home. Counting the number of words per hour addressed to children in the homes of professional families, working-class families, and families on public assistance, they extrapolated that by the time children were 4 years old, advantaged children had roughly 30 million more words addressed to them than the least advantaged–a finding replicated and often referred to as the "30 million word gap" [59,61,62]. A recent study by Amy Pace and her colleagues found that a child's language competency in kindergarten predicts later language, math, reading, and social abilities up to fifth grade and is the best early indicator of success [63]. Because language is so important as a foundation for learning, teaching families how to talk early and often to their children is the type of guidance that FNPs and all child health providers need to be offering to parents at their well-child visits.

Home language

Culture shapes all our experiences, and there can be profound differences across cultures in the way parents raise their children. The cultural lens influences how people think, interact, and view others. One of the areas in which cultural variation is most evident is the way in which parents talk with their children. As child health providers, it is important to acknowledge those differences and encourage families to adopt a more "conversational" style with their babies, to foster reciprocity in the communication. More and more children in the US come from homes where a language other than English is spoken [64]. The term "dual language learner" is used to refer to children who are

Table 2
Online resources for providers

Organization	Website

CDC: Learn the Signs. Act Early
  Free research-based, parent-friendly re-
  sources to assist health care providers
  with developmental surveillance from
  age 2 mo to 5 y.
	https://www.cdc.gov/ncbddd/actearly/
	  milestones/index.html

Parents as Teachers
  Parents are children's first teachers, and this
  site offers parenting tips and information.
	https://parentsasteachers.org/

Zero to Three
  Parent and professional resource for child
  development from birth to 3 y.
	http://www.zerotothree.org

Bright Futures Guidelines for Health
Supervision of Infants, Children, and
Adolescents
  Detailed information on well-child care for
  health care practitioners. This includes
  recommendations on providing antici-
  patory guidance and screening for de-
  lays in social-emotional development.
	https://brightfutures.aap.org/materials-and-
	  tools/guidelines-and-pocket-guide/Pages/
	  default.aspx

The Resilience Project
  This project is designed to provide
  resources for pediatricians and medical
  home teams to more effectively identify
  and care for children and adolescents
  who have been exposed to violence.
	https://www.aap.org/en-us/advocacy-and-
	  policy/aap-health-initiatives/resilience/
	  Pages/Resilience-Project.aspx

Reach out and Read
  The AAP officially endorsed the Reach Out
  and Read model of early literacy
  promotion.
	http://www.reachoutandread.org/

Read Conmigo ("Read With Me")
  Bilingual literacy program that provides
  free children's books in English and
  Spanish
	http://www.readconmigo.org/

Too Small to Fail & Talking is Teaching
  Public awareness and action campaign to
  promote the importance of early brain
  and language development and boost
  children's early brain and vocabulary
  development through simple, everyday
  actions
	http://toosmall.org/
	http://talkingisteaching.org

developing in their home language and in English and highlights their linguistic capacity in more than one language. Dual language learning is an opportunity for even greater language enrichment in children; therefore, the home language should be encouraged because it can foster greater acquisition in both languages as the child gets older [65]. Many families receive misinformed advice to switch to nonnative English with their children [66]. Contrary to the advice many immigrant families receive from trusted sources (including nurses, doctors, and teachers), linguistic research shows that nonnative language input is less useful for babies' language acquisition than high-quality native input. Scientific evidence consistently shows that teaching and encouraging bilingualism have positive outcomes for young children [67–72]. Of note, infants have the innate capacity to acquire 2 languages and can easily separate the sounds of each language [67]. There is no scientific evidence indicating that learning 2 languages during the early childhood years overwhelms, confuses, or significantly delays a child's acquisition of English [68]. Young bilingual children achieve critical milestones, such as babbling and onset of first words, within the same timeframe as typically developing monolingual children [69]. The reason for this is that home language provides a foundation for learning English—many skills developed in the first language transfer to the second. An extensive body of research highlights the many benefits that speaking more than one language has in many areas of development, including cognitive function [70–72]. It is imperative that FNPs understand how the science of home language can and should be applied to early childhood experiences to provide guidance and answer many of the questions that families will present with during their well-child visits.

Implications for practice

FNPs function in a broad variety of roles in the health care system: as clinicians, teachers, researchers, and advocates for patients across the lifespan. FNPs may see children during early childhood for routine well-child visits, during periods of acute illness or injury, or for chronic disease management. In any of these roles and settings where FNPs care for patients during early childhood, FNPs are ideally suited to provide a family-oriented approach and partner with parents and other important caregivers to design interventions and treatment plans to mitigate ACEs and to promote health, education, and literacy.

Caring for children during early childhood is a rewarding part of an FNP's scope of practice. FNPs who care for children during early childhood play a critical role in identifying that the child's health and development are a part of the family's development and functioning. In the face of many competing priorities during any outpatient visit, FNPs should remain grounded in a family-centered approach in order to develop interventions that are strengths-based and culturally sensitive, knowing that strong family support can help buffer the impact of psychosocial stressors.

This paper establishes the rationale for delivering health care to children and their families that transcends the conventional biomedical, anticipatory guidance model and embraces the assessment of the child in his or her community. Although there is good evidence from the AAP Bright Futures on using development screening tools such as the Modified Checklist for Autism in Toddlers and Ages and Stages Questionnaire, it is important to consider routinely posing questions about food insecurity, ACEs, stress, and trauma to inform the larger context of the child's growth and development (Table 3).

Table 3
Early childhood developmental/behavioral/social screening tools

	Sample available screening tools	AAP-recommended age
General Developmental Screening	• Ages and Stages Questionnaire (ASQ) • Parents' Evaluation of Developmental Status (PEDS) • Survey of Wellbeing of Young Children	9, 18, and 30 mo
Autism Spectrum Disorder Screening	• Modified Checklist for Autism in Toddlers • Survey of Wellbeing of Young Children (at specific ages)	18 and 24 mo
Social-Emotional Development	• Ages and Stages Questionnaire: Social-Emotional (ASQ-SE) • Pediatric Symptom Checklist (PSC) • Survey of Wellbeing of Young Children	"Regular intervals" depending on screening tool
Maternal Postpartum Depression	Edinburgh Postpartum Depression Scale (EPDS)	By 1 mo; then 2, 4, and 6 mo
Food Insecurity [27]	Hunger Vital Sign	At well-child visits
Social Determinants of Health	• A Safe Environment for Every Kid (SEEK) Questionnaire • Income, Transportation, Housing, Education, Legal Status, Literacy, and Personal Safety (IHELLP) • Protocol for Responding to and Assessing Patients' Assets, Risks, and Experiences (PRAPARE) • Well-Child Care, Evaluation, Community Resources, Advocacy, Referral, Education Survey Instrument (WE CARE) • Survey of Wellbeing of Young Children	Increasing focus in Bright Futures, but broad screening not yet specifically recommended
Adverse Childhood Experiences (ACEs)	• Center for Youth Wellness ACE Questionnaire (CYW ACE-Q) • Survey of Wellbeing of Young Children	Not yet specifically recommended

Data from Refs. [73–75]

Furthermore, by recognizing the synergistic relationship between health and education outcomes, FNPs can promote cognitive development and educational achievement by guiding families toward high-quality childcare options and encouraging language development and early literacy in the home. Given the documented benefits of ECE, FNPs can advocate for ECE environments that match the demand in the jurisdictions where they work. If developmental or behavioral concerns are identified by childcare providers, FNPs may contribute to the development of care plans for children in the childcare setting through consultation about treatment plans within the childcare setting and through initiating and maintaining contact with schools as appropriate. FNPs should encourage families to expose children to rich vocabulary in the home, even when the family's first language is not English.

FNPs who see patients during early childhood should cultivate child-friendly clinical environments where children and family members feel welcomed, respected, and valued. Siblings and important caregivers (eg, grandparents) may be invited to participate in visits as a way to recognize their role and contribution in the child's growth and development. Lastly, an important function of FNPs is to recognize when concerns that are identified warrant a referral to an appropriate specialist or community resource, including social services. FNPs should familiarize themselves with the network of resources in the areas where they practice and be prepared to collaborate with other professionals to support and empower families.

References

[1] Center on the Developing Child. Brain architecture. 2018. Available at: https://developingchild.harvard.edu/science/key-concepts/brain-architecture/. Accessed August 31, 2018.

[2] Lake A, Chan M. Putting science into practice for early child development. Lancet 2015;385(9980):1816–7.

[3] Hertzman C. The case for child development as a determinant of health. Can J Public Health 1998;89(Suppl 1):21.

[4] Kalmakis KA, Chandler GE. Health consequences of adverse childhood experiences: a systematic review. J Am Assoc Nurse Pract 2015;27(8):457–65.

[5] Shonkoff JP, Boyce WT, Cameron J, et al. Excessive stress disrupts the architecture of the developing brain: working paper 3 2014. Available at: http://www.developingchild.harvard.edu. Accessed August 31, 2018.

[6] Freed GL, Dunham KM, Loveland-Cherry C, et al. Family nurse practitioners: Roles and scope of practice in the care of pediatric patients. Pediatrics 2010;126(5):861–4.

[7] Webber E, Serowoky M. Breastfeeding curricular content of family nurse practitioner programs. J Pediatr Health Care 2017;31(2):189–95.

[8] Dixon DB, Kornblum AP, Steffen LM, et al. Implementation of lipid screening guidelines in children by primary pediatric providers. J Pediatr 2014;164(3):572–6.

[9] dela Cruz GG, Rozier RG, Slade G. Dental screening and referral of young children by pediatric primary care providers. Pediatrics 2004;114(5):642.

[10] Hornor G. Child maltreatment: screening and anticipatory guidance. J Pediatr Health Care 2013;27(4):242–50.

[11] Kim-Godwin Y, McMurry MJ. Perspectives of nurse practitioners on health care needs among latino children and families in the rural southeastern united states: A pilot study. J Pediatr Health Care 2012;26(6):409–17.

[12] Brady MA, Neal JA. Role delineation study of pediatric nurse practitioners: a national study of practice responsibilities and trends in role functions. J Pediatr Health Care 2000;14(4): 149–59.

[13] Shonkoff JP. Capitalizing on advances in science to reduce the health consequences of early childhood adversity. JAMA Pediatr 2016;170(10):1003–7.

[14] Centers for Disease Control and Prevention. Social determinants of health. 2018. Available at: https://www.cdc.gov/socialdeterminants/. Accessed August 21, 2018.

[15] Centers for Disease Control and Prevention. CDC research on SDOH. 2017. Available at: https://www.cdc.gov/socialdeterminants/research/index.htm. Accessed August 21, 2018.

[16] United States Census Bureau. Income and poverty in the United States: 2016. 2017. Available at: https://www.census.gov/library/publications/2017/demo/p60-259.html. Accessed August 21, 2018.

[17] Council on Community Pediatrics. Poverty and child health in the united states. Pediatrics 2016;137(4). Available at: https://pediatrics.aappublications.org/content/137/4/e20160339. Accessed August 21, 2018.

[18] Felitti VJ, Anda RF, Nordenberg D, et al. Relationship of childhood abuse and household dysfunction to many of the leading causes of death in adults. the adverse childhood experiences (ACE) study. Am J Prev Med 1998;14(4):245–58.

[19] Bethell CD, Carle A, Hudziak J, et al. Methods to assess adverse childhood experiences of children and families: Toward approaches to promote child well-being in policy and practice. Acad Pediatr 2017;17(7):S69.

[20] Barth RP, Scarborough A, Lloyd EC, et al. Developmental status and early intervention service needs of maltreated children. 2008. Available at: https://files.eric.ed.gov/fulltext/ED501753.pdf. Accessed August 31, 2018.

[21] Sacks V, Murphey D. The prevalence of adverse childhood experiences, nationally, by state, and by race or ethnicity. 2018. Available at: https://www.childtrends.org/publications/prevalence-adverse-childhood-experiences-nationally-state-race-ethnicity. Accessed August 19, 2018.

[22] Garner AS, Shonkoff JP. Early childhood adversity, toxic stress, and the role of the pediatrician: translating developmental science into lifelong health. Pediatrics 2012;129:e224.

[23] American Academy of Pediatrics. The resilience project: clinical assessment tools. 2018. Available at: https://www.aap.org/en-us/advocacy-and-policy/aap-health-initiatives/resilience/Pages/Clinical-Assessment-Tools.aspx. Accessed August 21, 2018.

[24] Cohen JA, Kelleher KJ, Mannarino AP. Identifying, treating, and referring traumatized children: the role of pediatric providers. Arch Pediatr Adolesc Med 2008;162(5):447–52.

[25] Brcic V, Eberdt C, Kaczorowski J. Development of a tool to identify poverty in a family practice setting: a pilot study. Int J Fam Med 2011;2011:812182.

[26] Garg A, Butz AM, Dworkin PH, et al. Improving the management of family psychosocial problems at low-income children's well-child care visits: the WE CARE project. Pediatrics 2007;120(3):547–58.

[27] Council on Community Pediatrics, Committee on Nutrition. Promoting food security for all children. Pediatrics 2015;136(5):1431. Available at: https://pediatrics.aappublications.org/content/136/5/e1431. Accessed August 22, 2018.

[28] Hager ER, Quigg AM, Black MM, et al. Development and validity of a 2-item screen to identify families at risk for food insecurity. Pediatrics 2010;126(1):e26–32.

[29] Johnson SB, Riley AW, Granger DA, et al. The science of early life toxic stress for pediatric practice and advocacy. Pediatrics 2013;131(2):319–27.

[30] Peacock-Chambers E, Ivy K, Bair-Merritt M. Primary care interventions for early childhood development: A systematic review. Pediatrics 2017;140(6) [pii:e20171661].

[31] Purewal Boparai SK, Au V, Koita K, et al. Ameliorating the biological impacts of childhood adversity: a review of intervention programs. Child Abuse Negl 2018;81:82–105.

[32] Youssef NA, Belew D, Hao G, et al. Racial/ethnic differences in the association of child-hood adversities with depression and the role of resilience. J Affect Disord 2017;208: 577–81.

[33] Duursma E, Augustyn M, Zuckerman B. Reading aloud to children: the evidence. Arch Dis Child 2008;93(7):554–7.

[34] Willis E, Kabler-Babbitt C, Zuckerman B. Early literacy interventions: reach out and read. Pediatr Clin North Am 2007;54(3):625–42.

[35] Council on Community Pediatrics. The role of preschool home-visiting programs in improving children's developmental and health outcomes. Pediatrics 2009;123(2):598–603.

[36] Shonkoff JP, Boyce WT, McEwen BS. Neuroscience, molecular biology, and the childhood roots of health disparities: building a new framework for health promotion and disease pre-vention. JAMA 2009;301(21):2252–9.

[37] Anderson LM, Shinn C, Fullilove MT, et al. The effectiveness of early childhood development programs. A systematic review. Am J Prev Med 2003;24(3 Suppl):32–46.

[38] Bakken L, Brown N, Downing B. Early childhood education: the long-term benefits. J Res Child Educ 2017;31(2):255–69.

[39] Sick N, Spaulding S, Park Y. Understanding young-parent families. 2018. Available at: https://www.urban.org/research/publication/understanding-young-parent-families. Ac-cessed August 31, 2018.

[40] Mackenzie S, Evers S. Identifying concerns of parents of young children. Can Fam Physician 1986;32:1281–4.

[41] Paschall K, Trout K. Most child care settings in the united states are homes, not centers. Child Trends 2018. Available at: https://www.childtrends.org/most-child-care-providers-in-the-united-states-are-based-in-homes-not-centers. Accessed August 31, 2018.

[42] Donoghue EA. Quality early education and child care from birth to kindergarten. Pediatrics 2017;140(2) [pii: e20171488]. Available at: http://pediatrics.aappublications.org/con-tent/140/2/e20171488.long. Accessed August 31, 2018.

[43] Nores M, Belfield CR, Barnett WS, et al. Updating the economic impacts of the high/scope perry preschool program. Educ Eval Policy Anal 2005;27(3):245–61. Available at: https://www.jstor.org/stable/3699571. Accessed August 31, 2018.

[44] Campbell F, Conti G, Heckman JJ, et al. Early childhood investments substantially boost adult health. Science 2014;343(6178):1478–85.

[45] Community Preventive Services Task Force. Promoting health equity through education pro-grams and policies: Center-based early childhood education. 2016. Available at: https://www.thecommunityguide.org/sites/default/files/assets/Health-Equity-Center-Based-Early-Childhood-Education_3.pdf. Accessed September 2, 2018.

[46] Augustine JM, Crosnoe RL, Gordon R. Early child care and illness among preschoolers. J Health Soc Behav 2013;54(3):315–34.

[47] Gilliam WS, Yale University Child Study Center. Prekindergarteners left behind: expulsion rates in state prekindergarten systems. 2005. Available at: https://www.fcd-us.org/as-sets/2016/04/ExpulsionCompleteReport.pdf. Accessed September 2, 2018.

[48] US Department of Education Office for Civil Rights. Civil rights data collection data snap-shot: early childhood education. 2014. Available at: https://www2.ed.gov/about/of-fices/list/ocr/docs/crdc-early-learning-snapshot.pdf. Accessed August 31, 2018.

[49] Gilliam W, Maupin A, Reyes C, et al. Do early educators' implicit biases regarding sex and race relate to behavior expectations and recommendations of preschool expulsions and sus-pensions?. 2016. Available at: https://medicine.yale.edu/childstudy/zigler/publications/Preschool%20Implicit%20Bias%20Policy%20Brief_final_9_26_276766_5379_v1.pdf. Ac-cessed August 31, 2018.

[50] Project Implicit. Implicit association test. 2017. Available at: https://implicit.harvard.edu/implicit/. Accessed August 31, 2018.

[51] Head Zauche L, Thul TA, Darcy Mahoney AE, et al. Influence of language nutrition on children's language and cognitive development: an integrated review. Early Child Res Q 2016;36:318–33.

[52] Hoff E. Interpreting the early language trajectories of children from low-SES and language minority homes: Implications for closing achievement gaps. Dev Psychol 2013;49(1):4–14.

[53] Head Zauche L, Darcy Mahoney AE, Thul TA, et al. The power of language nutrition for children's brain development, health, and future academic achievement. J Pediatr Health Care 2017;31(4):493–503. Available at: https://www.clinicalkey.es/playcontent/1-s2.0-S089152451630311X.

[54] Rowe ML. A longitudinal investigation of the role of quantity and quality of child-directed speech in vocabulary development. Child Development 2012;83(5):1762–74.

[55] Dickinson DK, Porche MV. Relation between language experiences in preschool classrooms and children's kindergarten and fourth-grade language and reading abilities. Child Dev 2011;82(3):870–86.

[56] Durham R, Farkas G, Hammer C, et al. Kindergarten oral language skill: a key variable in the intergenerational transmission of socioeconomic status. Res Soc Stratif Mob 2007;25: 294–305.

[57] Rowe ML, Raudenbush SW, Goldin-Meadow S. The pace of vocabulary growth helps predict later vocabulary skill. Child Dev 2012;83(2):508–25.

[58] Weisleder A, Fernald A. Talking to children matters. Psychol Sci 2013;24(11):2143–52.

[59] Weldon, AB. Language Nutrition: filling the word opportunity gap. Speech given at the National Meeting of State Leads for the National Campaign for Grade-Level Reading. Washington, DC. January 9, 2014.

[60] The Nation's Report Card. NAEP report cards - home. 2018. Available at: https://www.nationsreportcard.gov/. Accessed September 2, 2018.

[61] Golinkoff RM, Hoff E, Rowe M, et al. Talking with children matters: defending the 30 million word gap. 2018. Available at: https://www.brookings.edu/blog/education-plus-development/2018/05/21/defending-the-30-million-word-gap-disadvantaged-children-dont-hear-enough-child-directed-words/. Accessed September 2, 2018.

[62] Hart B, Risley TR. Meaningful differences in the everyday experience of young American children. Baltimore (MD): Brookes; 1995.

[63] Pace A, Alper R, Burchinal MR, et al. Measuring success: Within and cross-domain predictors of academic and social trajectories in elementary school. Early Child Res Q 2019;46: 112–25.

[64] Children's Defense Fund. The state of America's children 2017 report. 2017. Available at: https://www.childrensdefense.org/reports/2017/the-state-of-americas-children-2017-report/. Accessed Sep 2, 2018.

[65] Talk with me baby 2.0. Available at: http://www.talkwithmebaby.org/. Accessed September 2, 2018.

[66] Montrul S. El bilingüismo en el mundo hispanohablante. Malden (MA): Wiley-Blackwell; 2013.

[67] Conboy BT, Kuhl PK. Impact of second-language experience in infancy: Brain measures of first- and second-language speech perception. Dev Sci 2011;14(2):242–8.

[68] Espinosa L. Getting it RIGHT for young children from diverse backgrounds: applying research to improve practice with a focus on dual language learners. 2nd edition. New York: Pearson; 2015.

[69] Paradis J, Nicoladis E, Crago M, et al. Bilingual children's acquisition of the past tense: a usage-based approach. J Child Lang 2011;38(3):554–78.

[70] Head LM, Baralt M, Darcy Mahoney AE. Bilingualism as a potential strategy to improve executive function in preterm infants: a review. J Pediatr Health Care 2015;29(2):126–36.

[71] Bialystok E. Bilingualism in development: language, literacy, and cognition. Cambridge (United Kingdom): Cambridge University Press; 2001.

[72] National Head Start Training and Technical Assistance Research Center. Dual language learning: What does it take? Head Start dual language report. 2008. Available at: http://www.buildinitiative.org/Portals/0/Uploads/Documents/Dual%20Language%20Learning%20-%20What%20Does%20It%20Take.pdf. Accessed September 2, 2018.

[73] American Academy of Pediatrics. Screening recommendations. 2018. Available at: https://www.aap.org/en-us/advocacy-and-policy/aap-health-initiatives/Screening/Pages/Screening-Recommendations.aspx. Accessed September 2, 2018.

[74] American Academy of Pediatrics. Screening tools. 2017. Available at: https://screening-time.org/star-center/#/screening-tools. Accessed September 2, 2018.

[75] American Academy of Pediatrics. Periodicity schedule. 2018. Available at: https://www.aap.org/en-us/professional-resources/practice-transformation/managing-patients/Pages/Periodicity-Schedule.aspx. Accessed September 2, 2018.

Advances in Family Practice Nursing 1 (2019) 201–210

ADVANCES IN FAMILY PRACTICE NURSING

Transition of Health Care in Children with Chronic Health Conditions

Sharron Close, PhD, MS, CPNP-PC[a,b,*],
Susan Brasher, PhD, MS, CPNP-PC[a],
Amy Blumling, RN, CPNP-PC[a], Amy Talboy, MD[b],
Kristy Martyn, PhD, CPNP-PC[a]

[a]Nell Hodgson Woodruff School of Nursing, 1520 Clifton Road NE # 434, Atlanta, GA 30322, USA; [b]Department of Human Genetics, eXtraordinarY Clinic, Emory School of Medicine, 1365 Clifton Road, Northeast, Suite 2200, Atlanta, GA 30322, USA

Keywords
- Transition of health care • Chronic conditions • Model of transitional care
- Pediatric to adult • Continuity of care

Key points
- Chronic conditions beginning in childhood often persist into adulthood requiring systematic health surveillance and special considerations for continuity of care.
- As children with chronic conditions grow toward maturity, multifactorial needs must be addressed in the pediatric setting with the goal of achieving self-management in the adult health care setting.
- Family nurse practitioners can play a key role in achieving positive health outcomes for children with chronic conditions by using a systematic and coordinated transition of care approach in the primary care setting.

INTRODUCTION

Assisting children and their families in transitioning from pediatric health care to adult health care involves preparing patients and families to become involved in understanding their own health status, anticipation of current

Disclosure: S. Close, S. Brasher, A. Blumling, A. Talboy, and K. Martyn have nothing to disclose.

*Corresponding author. Nell Hodgson Woodruff School of Nursing, 1520 Clifton Road NE # 434, Atlanta, GA 30322. E-mail address: sharron.m.close@emory.edu

https://doi.org/10.1016/j.yfpn.2019.01.004
2589-420X/19/© 2019 Elsevier Inc. All rights reserved.

and future health needs, and active engagement with health care providers. The process requires systematic transition planning that takes a comprehensive look at health care needs in the context of developmental and psychosocial needs of the child [1,2]. Since the mid to late 1990s, the need for transition from pediatric to adult health care services has been cited in the literature as a fundamental part of providing continuity of care for all children and especially those with chronic health conditions [2–6]. However, implementing a plan for transition of care can be an overlooked or challenging process in primary health care delivery. When adolescents and young adults (AYAs) approach the age of 18 years, many are ill-prepared to assume the responsibility of taking over their own health maintenance requirements. This unpreparedness may, in part, be caused by an extended dependence on parents and family as young adults venture into higher education, vocational training, or first-jobs. As well, many AYAs are in stages of development known for feeling powerful, independent, and sometimes invincible against a background of immaturity and willingness to be exposed to health risks. Once leaving home and leaving the regular care of a pediatric health care provider, many young adults forgo regular health maintenance and, instead, seek health care in the case of illness or injury only. Without systematic health maintenance, health screening, and anticipatory health guidance, good health status is at risk. This gap in care invites continuation of potentially unhealthy behaviors and missed opportunities to intervene. Without preventive health care, maintenance AYAs are at risk of poor health outcomes.

Children with chronic conditions that are well managed while living at home represent a special at-risk group when they become AYAs [7]. Without specialized, coordinated, and often multidisciplinary care, children with chronic diseases become adults with multiple chronic conditions that complicate their life course with significant physical and psychosocial comorbidities. Approximately one-third of adults around the world now live with more than 1 chronic condition, resulting in a high burden of poor health outcomes and high health costs, and this is expected to increase dramatically [8,9]. Planning for transition from pediatric to adult health care is an essential step in bridging an important health care delivery gap that offers improvement in individual as well as population health. This article discusses evidence that supports why transition planning is important for continuity of care and how patient health outcomes can be influenced for the better. Guidance for implementing a health care transition approach into practice and resources for family nurse practitioners (FNPs) and primary care providers (PCPs) is also offered.

LIFETIME CHRONIC HEALTH CONDITIONS BEGINNING IN CHILDHOOD

How chronic conditions or diseases are defined complicates how clinicians think about, study, and care for children who have complex conditions requiring ongoing care. According to the US National Center for Health

Statistics, 27% of children in the United States have a chronic condition and, of those, 1 in 15 have multiple chronic conditions [10]. A few of the more common chronic conditions beginning in childhood include asthma, allergies, diabetes, obesity/overweight, inflammatory bowel disease/Crohn disease, developmental disabilities such as attention-deficit/hyperactivity disorder and autism, and some mental health issues [11]. Some conditions of genetic derivation, such as cystic fibrosis and sickle cell disease, are also widely recognized as chronic, whereas others are not. The many disparate descriptions of how the term chronic disease is defined are shown in Table 1. Left out of formal consideration as chronic disease are several other conditions, including those of genetic origin that manifest symptoms and problems in childhood requiring specialized lifelong health surveillance, treatment, and services through adulthood. Genetic conditions such as Down syndrome, Fragile X, and persons born with X and Y chromosome variations are just a few of those examples. Genetic conditions with chronic comorbidities often involve complex care to manage physical and psychosocial issues. Healthy children and those with chronic conditions will always require systematic primary care, even though some of them may require the attention of specialists. FNPs and PCPs play an important role in educating, coordinating, and planning for lifespan care for patients with chronic conditions and those that are or not formally recognized as chronic conditions.

PERSPECTIVE OF HEALTH CARE TRANSITION FOR FAMILY NURSE PRACTITIONERS

FNPs and PCPs are prepared to care for medically stable patients across the lifespan from infants to geriatric patients in primary or specialty practice settings. Because FNPs are expected to care for individuals throughout the lifespan, an argument might be made for why pediatric-to-adult health care transition should be an issue for consideration in practice. Although the FNP scope of practice includes the lifespan approach, many FNPs specialize within the context of primary care, frequently focusing on adults, geriatrics, women's health, and sometimes within specialties such as cancer and palliative care. However, FNPs may find themselves receiving new young patients for the first time who have previously received primary care in the pediatric setting. For transitioning young patients with chronic conditions needing primary care, FNPs are well positioned to partner with patients and families in the coordination and delivery of a new care plan that takes developmental trajectory into account.

POSITIVE OUTCOMES FROM STRUCTURED TRANSITION OF CARE

A recent systematic review by Gabriel and colleagues [12] focused on studies that examined structured pediatric-to-adult health care transition interventions. Out of 43 studies reviewed, 28 showed positive outcomes. Although these outcomes were not solely focused on clinical parameters, they contribute combined

Table 1
Disparate definitions of chronic disease

Source	Definition	
CDC	Chronic diseases are defined broadly as conditions that last 1 y or more and require ongoing medical attention, or limit activities of daily living, or both. Chronic diseases such as heart disease, cancer, and diabetes are the leading causes of death and disability in the United States	
NIH	Chronic medical conditions, including cardiovascular disease, cancer, diabetes, and depression, cause more than half of all deaths worldwide	
WHO	Diseases that are not passed from person to person. They are of long duration and, generally, slow progression. The 4 main types are cardiovascular diseases (eg, heart attacks and stroke), cancers, chronic respiratory diseases (eg, chronic obstructed pulmonary disease and asthma), and diabetes	
Centers for Medicare and Medicaid Services	Alzheimer disease and related dementia	Heart failure
	Arthritis (osteoarthritis and rheumatoid)	Hepatitis (chronic viral B and C)
	Asthma	HIV/AIDS
	Atrial fibrillation	Hyperlipidemia (high cholesterol level)
	Autism spectrum disorders	Hypertension (high blood pressure)
	Cancer (breast, colorectal, lung, and prostate)	Ischemic Heart Disease
	Chronic kidney disease	Osteoporosis
	Chronic obstructive pulmonary disease	Schizophrenia and other psychotic disorders
	Depression	Stroke
	Diabetes	—
US National Center for Health Statistics	One lasting 3 mo or more, by the definition of the US National Center for Health Statistics. Chronic diseases generally cannot be prevented by vaccines or cured by medication, nor do they just disappear	

Abbreviations: AIDS, acquired immunodeficiency syndrome; CDC, US centers for disease control and prevention; HIV, human immunodeficiency virus; NIH, National Institutes of Health; WHO, World Health Organization.

evidence that supports benefits in population health, consumer experience, and reduction in transition barriers. Positive service use impacts were shown in 9 of the studies with no significant cost savings reported out of 3 studies that examined cost. Systematic reviews, by method, also evaluated studies in terms of strength of evidence. Quality of evidence was assessed by an evaluation instrument known as the Effective Public Health Practice Quality Assessment Tool for Quantitative Studies. Note that 7 studies (16%) were rated as methodologically strong, with 18 (42%) rated as moderate and 18 (42%) rated as weak. These strength-of-evidence ratings show that future interventions and intervention studies need to focus improvements on methods and, perhaps, on finding common core elements of variables that make comparisons between interventions and between studies more meaningful. Nevertheless, it must be kept in mind that professional organizations such as the American Academy of Pediatrics (AAP), the American Academy of Family Practitioners (AAFP), and the American College of Physicians (ACP) only recently recommended a structured transition process with steps for transition planning and transfer with integration to adult care [6]. These recommendations have yet to be widely adopted into practice.

GENERAL HEALTH CARE TRANSITION PLANNING IN PEDIATRICS

Studies have shown that transition preparation and implementation are lacking for children with special health care needs [13,14]. As a result, they are vulnerable to discontinuity of care [15], delays and gaps in finding primary and specialty care [16], issues with treatment and medication adherence [17], and poor health outcomes [18]. In 2011, a joint clinical report was prepared by the AAP, the AAFP, and the ACP calling for specific clinical intervention beginning at 12 years of age through young adulthood [6]. In 2014, the National Academy of Medicine recognized that the transition of health care from pediatric to adult health care providers was a persistent problem with little evidence of systematic implementation and evaluation. The National Association of Pediatric Nurse Practitioners published a position statement in 2016 communicating that all pediatric health care providers should collaborate in providing pediatric health care medical homes with interventions that promote family-centered partnerships within communities and provide for transitional care from pediatric to adult services [19].

GOT TRANSITION BY THE AMERICAN ACADEMY OF PEDIATRICS

The Got Transition program [6] was created for use by pediatric, family medicine, combined internal Medicine & Pediatrics and, internal medicine health care providers, including advanced practice nurses. The program incorporates 6 core elements to provide structure and process for planning and implementation of successful transition. The 6 core elements are having a transition policy, developing a transition and tracking and monitoring process, conducting evaluation of readiness for transition, transition planning, transfer of care, and transfer completion.

Transition policy development begins within the FNP practice where clinicians and staff create a policy statement in collaboration with patients and families to explain that, beginning at age 12 years, care will involve teaching the adolescents about the need to understand their special health needs. They will be taught and given tools to help them establish reliable and systematic care so that, when they leave home, they will have confidence in how to care for themselves.

Transition tracking and monitoring is also a process to be established by the FNP practice to document and track the individual stages of transition from readiness to planning and transfer. This process may be incorporated through the electronic medical record system or by using flow sheets or electronic data tools.

Readiness evaluation is a systematic practice recommended to begin for patients at age 14 years that identifies needs and goals associated with self-care. Pediatric patients, caregivers, and the FNP partner as a team to map a plan for how the child/adolescent will move toward independent health decisions and self-care.

Transition planning involves maintaining an up-to-date plan of care, goals, routine and emergency care plans, and fact sheets, teaching about medical privacy and consent, including how to initiate release of medical information. This stage is also the time to introduce any new members of the adult-oriented health care provider team as well as providing resources regarding insurance coverages.

Transfer of care is the hand-off of care to the adult-oriented provider. It involves preparing a package of health care summary and goals, and identifying and introducing the health care provider who is taking over. Transfer may also involve consulting in tandem while the patient becomes established with the new adult provider.

Transfer completion is a final step when the pediatric provider elicits feedback in 3 to 6 months from the patient and the new provider on satisfaction and effectiveness of the transfer of care.

The 6 steps outlined in Got Transition represent frames of planning that can be adjusted according to patient preference and the practice philosophy.

HEALTH CARE TRANSITION FOR CHILDREN WITH CHRONIC CONDITIONS AND SPECIAL HEALTH CARE NEEDS

Patient-centered and family-centered care is vitally important to achieving optimum health management of children with chronic conditions and special health care needs. The concept of health is intricately intertwined with aspects of children's lives and development that are influenced by and directly affect health. Fig. 1 shows 7 key areas of transitions set against the background of complexities to be considered in chronic conditions. The 7 areas are daily living, education, job/career, self-advocacy, social life, safety and health systems, and payors. These areas represent breadth and complexity of considerations in the care of children with chronic conditions who become adults with chronic conditions. Fig. 1 also shows the continuum of the transitions process beginning at age 12 years and progressing through young adulthood.

GUIDANCE FOR IMPLEMENTATION INTO PRACTICE

Busy FNPs are likely to inquire about how to realistically incorporate 6 core elements of transition as described by the AAP along with 7 key areas of transition. Implementation of this manner of practice requires organization and coordination. One of the next emerging questions might be concerned with time spent and compensation. MacManus and colleagues [21] (2018) developed a

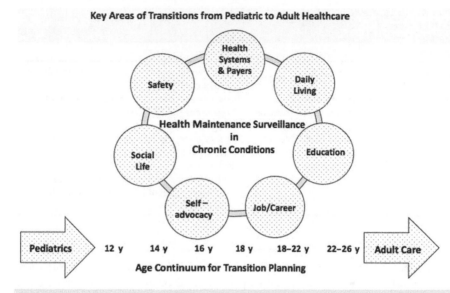

Fig. 1. Areas of health care transition in chronic disease across the age continuum. *Adapted from* Brasher S, Close S, Stapel-Wax J, et al. Engaging patients and stakeholders in a patient-centered outcomes research institute (PCORI) award to address transitioning to adulthood in autism spectrum disorder (ASD). Poster presented at the Academy Health Annual Research Meeting, Seattle, Washington, June 24–26, 2018.[20]

coding and reimbursement tip sheet for use when spending clinical time on the transition from pediatric to adult health care. This reference provides billable codes for clinical activities that include screening for transition readiness, chronic care management, education, and planning of patient self-management. For FNPs, the Got Transition 6 core elements provide structure for how to set up a transition program and also offer insight about the patient experience if the FNP is the adult provider receiving the hand-off from a pediatric provider. Implementation of any new program into clinical practice requires willingness to try, time to adjust, and patience to adopt something new. Success may also depend on consensus of the practitioners and staff that a program like this has value to both the patient and the practice.

DISCUSSION

Children with chronic conditions require effective primary and specialty care to optimize their growth and development and to shepherd them on to living their optimal lives. Transition of health care services and health care providers is a complex process that requires investment of time and effort for patients, families, and health care providers. When health care transition is done poorly, the patient is at risk of losing quality of care and access to care as well [22,23]. Several barriers to implementing pediatric-to-adult transition have

Table 2
Resources health care transitioning

Source	Web site
American Academy of Pediatrics Got Transition	https://www.gottransition.org/youthfamilies/index.cfm?
American Academy of Pediatrics ECHO (Virtual Training for Implementation of Healthcare Transition Planning)	https://www.aap.org/en-us/professional-resources/practice-transformation/echo/Pages/Transition.aspx
National Association of Pediatric Nurse Practitioners Position Statement	https://www.jpedhc.org/article/S0891-5245(15)00369-7/pdf
American College of Physicians	https://www.acponline.org/clinical-information/high-value-care/resources-for-clinicians/pediatric-to-adult-care-transitions-initiative

been identified. Some patients and families have difficulty moving on from their long-standing relationships with their pediatricians or may have negative beliefs about adult care [24]. Other barriers include access to insurance, limited patient and caregiver knowledge about medication, illness, or the need to plan for transition [25]. Overcoming barriers like these begins with systematic planning well in advance of transfer of care during the early adolescent years [26]. Transitioning must be customized according to patient need and according to the capacity of health care providers to implement plans that work in each practice setting. No one-size-fits-all option works in every circumstance. A number of useful websites to inform FNPs about resources in healthcare transitioning is summarized in Table 2.

SUMMARY
Because of advances in treatment, the landscape of chronic disease is changing. Children who might not have survived into adulthood in the past are now living lives well into adulthood while managing complex and sometimes multiple chronic conditions. FNPs and other health care providers can optimize care by providing anticipatory guidance, structure, and plans for smooth transition from pediatric to adult models of care. There is widespread agreement about the need for transition programs with no standard way of implementing or evaluating them. Using all or part of a program such as Got Transition by the AAP provides a place to begin with structure and resources that will benefit patients and families.

Acknowledgments
The author received Patient-Centered Research Institute Grant for (1) Bidirectional Translation of Knowledge and Need in Sex Chromosome Aneuploidies and (2) Engaging Patients and Stakeholders to Address Transitioning to Adulthood in Autism Spectrum Disorder.

References

[1] Mahan JD, Betz CL, Okumura MJ, et al. Self-management and transition to adult health care in adolescents and young adults: a team process. Pediatr Rev 2017;38(7):305–19.

[2] Betz CL. Transition of adolescents with special health care needs: review and analysis of the literature. Issues Compr Pediatr Nurs 2004;27(3):179–241.

[3] Betz CL, Redcay G. Lessons learned from providing transition services to adolescents with special health care needs. Issues Compr Pediatr Nurs 2002;25(2):129–49.

[4] American Academy of Pediatrics, American Academy of Family Physicians, American College of Physicians-American Society of Internal Medicine. A consensus statement on health care transitions for young adults with special health care needs. Pediatrics 2002;110(6 Pt 2):1304–6.

[5] Betz CL. Facilitating the transition of adolescents with chronic conditions from pediatric to adult health care and community settings. Issues Compr Pediatr Nurs 1998;21(2):97–115.

[6] American Academy of Pediatrics, American Academy of Family Physicians, American College of Physicians, Transitions Clinical Report Authoring Group, Cooley WC, Sagerman PJ. Supporting the health care transition from adolescence to adulthood in the medical home. Pediatrics 2011;128(1):182–200.

[7] Maeng DD, Snyder SR, Davis TW, et al. Impact of a complex care management model on cost and utilization among adolescents and young adults with special care and health needs. Popul Health Manag 2017;20(6):435–41.

[8] Buttorff C, Ruder T, Bauman M. Multiple chronic conditions in the United States. Santa Monica (CA): RAND Corporation; 2017. Available at: https://www.rand.org/pubs/tools/TL221.html. Accessed November 11, 2018.

[9] Marengoni A, Angleman S, Fratiglioni L. Prevalence of disability according to multimorbidity and disease clustering: a population-based study. J Comorb 2011;1:11–8.

[10] CDC National Center for Health Statistics. Tables of summary health statistics. 2018. Available at: https://www.cdc.gov/nchs/nhis/SHS/tables.htm. Accessed November 11, 2018.

[11] Torpy JM, Campbell A, Glass RM. JAMA patient page. Chronic diseases of children. JAMA 2010;303(7):682.

[12] Gabriel P, McManus M, Rogers K, et al. Outcome evidence for structured pediatric to adult health care transition interventions: a systematic review. J Pediatr 2017;188:263–269 e215.

[13] McManus MA, Pollack LR, Cooley WC, et al. Current status of transition preparation among youth with special needs in the United States. Pediatrics 2013;131(6):1090–7.

[14] Betz CL, Lobo ML, Nehring WM, et al. Voices not heard: a systematic review of adolescents' and emerging adults' perspectives of health care transition. Nurs Outlook 2013;61(5):311–36.

[15] Montano CB, Young J. Discontinuity in the transition from pediatric to adult health care for patients with attention-deficit/hyperactivity disorder. Postgrad Med 2012;124(5):23–32.

[16] Garvey K, Laffel L. Transitions in care from pediatric to adult health care providers: ongoing challenges and opportunities for young persons with diabetes. Endocr Dev 2018;33:68–81.

[17] Pai AL, Schwartz LA. Introduction to the special section: health care transitions of adolescents and young adults with pediatric chronic conditions. J Pediatr Psychol 2011;36(2):129–33.

[18] Annunziato RA, Emre S, Shneider B, et al. Adherence and medical outcomes in pediatric liver transplant recipients who transition to adult services. Pediatr Transplant 2007;11(6):608–14.

[19] NAPNAP position statement. Position statement on pediatric health care/medical home: key issues on care coordination, transitions, and leadership. J Pediatr Health Care 2016;30(2):A17–9.

[20] Brasher S, Close S, Stapel-Wax J, et al. Engaging patients and stakeholders in a patient-centered outcomes research institute (PCORI) award to address transitioning to adulthood

in autism spectrum disorder (ASD). Poster presented at the Academy Health Annual Research Meeting, Seattle, Washington, June 24–26, 2018.

[21] McManus M, White P, Schmidt A, et al. Coding and reimbursement tip sheet for transition from pediatric to adult health care. Washington, DC: National Alliance to Advance Adolescent Health; 2018. Available at: https://www.gottransition.org/resourceGet.cfm?id=352. Accessed November 28, 2018.

[22] Scal P, Davern M, Ireland M, et al. Transition to adulthood: delays and unmet needs among adolescents and young adults with asthma. J Pediatr 2008;152(4):471–5, 475.e1.

[23] Okumura MJ, Hersh AO, Hilton JF, et al. Change in health status and access to care in young adults with special health care needs: results from the 2007 National Survey of Adult Transition and Health. J Adolesc Health 2013;52(4):413–8.

[24] Gray WN, Schaefer MR, Resmini-Rawlinson A, et al. Barriers to transition from pediatric to adult care: a systematic review. J Pediatr Psychol 2018;43(5):488–502.

[25] Cope R, Jonkman L, Quach K, et al. Transitions of care: medication-related barriers identified by low socioeconomic patients of a federally qualified health center following hospital discharge. Res Social Adm Pharm 2018;14(1):26–30.

[26] Goralski JL, Nasr SZ, Uluer A. Overcoming barriers to a successful transition from pediatric to adult care. Pediatr Pulmonol 2017;52(S48):S52–60.

Advances in Family Practice Nursing 1 (2019) 211–218

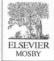

ADVANCES IN FAMILY PRACTICE NURSING

ELSEVIER
MOSBY

Immunization Schedule Updates for Children, Adolescents, and Adults

Kimberly R. Joo, DNP, APRN-CNP, CNE, EBP-C

The Ohio State University, College of Nursing, Dayton Children's Hospital, Springboro Urgent Care, Kids Express, 377 Newton Hall, 1585 Neil Avenue, Columbus, OH 43210, USA

Keywords
- Vaccination schedule • Immunization schedule • Pediatric • Children • Adolescent
- Adult • 2019 immunization update • 2019 vaccination update

Key points
- The immunization schedules for children and adolescents and adults more than 18 years of age were updated in February of 2019.
- Key recommendation changes for children and adolescents schedule in 2019 included influenza, hepatitis A, hepatitis B, inactivated polio vaccine, tetanus, diphtheria, and pertussis (Tdap) vaccines, and recommendations for outbreaks.
- Key recommendation changes for the adult schedule in 2019 included influenza, hepatitis A, and hepatitis B vaccines.

INTRODUCTION

The Advisory Committee on Immunization Practices (ACIP) develops recommendations for immunization schedules for children, adolescents, and adults. This committee is composed of medical and public health experts who meet 3 times a year to review current vaccine research findings and scientific data regarding the safe and effective use of vaccines, clinical trial results, and manufacturer's labeling and package inserts [1]. The most recent recommendations were approved in October of 2018 and were published in February 2019. The immunization schedules released in 2019 were titled Recommended Child and Adolescent Immunization Schedule for Ages 18 Years or Younger, 2019,

Disclosure: The author has no financial or commercial conflicts of interest to disclose.

E-mail address: joo.134@osu.edu

https://doi.org/10.1016/j.yfpn.2018.12.006

United States and Recommended Adult Immunization Schedule for Ages 19 Years or Older, 2019, United States. All recommendations were approved by ACIP, the American Academy of Pediatrics (AAP), the American Academy of Family Physicians (AAFP), and the American College of Obstetricians and Gynecologists (ACOG) [1].

BACKGROUND AND SIGNIFICANCE

The invention of vaccines has been named one of the 10 great public health achievements in the past several decades [2]. Before vaccines, infectious disease was a leading cause of death in both children and adults [3]. The prevention of disease is a key objective of vaccines. Each vaccine given to a child or an adult assists the body's own immune system to fight diseases through the development of antigens that provide immunity to a specific disease [4]. Immunizations prevent an estimated 42,000 deaths and avert 20 million new cases of disease each year. This prevention results in a net saving of close to $14 billion dollars [4]. The Centers for Disease Control and Prevention (CDC) tracks current immunization/vaccination rates in the United States. The most current data show an overall vaccination rate for children aged 19 to 35 months at 74.1% [5]. The most current vaccination rates for adolescents aged 13 to 17 years are tracked by specific vaccination. The best rates include hepatitis B (HepB) vaccine at 91.4% and measles, mumps, and rubella (MMR) at 90.9%. Middle-range rates were tetanus, diphtheria, and pertussis (Tdap) at 88%, varicella at 85.6%, and meningococcal at 82.2%. The lowest vaccination rates for adolescents were for the human papilloma virus. Female rates were 43% and male rates were 31.5% [6]. Vaccination rates for adults aged 18 years and older are only tracked for influenza and pneumococcal rates. The rate for influenza is 40.9% and the rate for pneumococcal is 22.9% [7,8].

This article provides a synopsis and explanation of the new 2019 changes to the adult and children and adolescent immunization schedules. The article reviews the changes to the children and adolescent immunization schedule followed by a review of the changes to the adult immunization schedule.

2019 CHANGES TO THE CHILDREN AND ADOLESCENTS IMMUNIZATION SCHEDULE

The immunization schedule for children and adolescents aged 18 years and younger includes a cover page, the recommended immunization schedule, the catch-up schedule, medical indications, and notes. The cover page includes a table of current vaccinations and combination vaccines with their abbreviation and trade names; directions on how to use the schedule; hyperlinks to the ACIP, CDC, AAP, ACOG Web sites; and hyperlinks to the Vaccine Adverse Event Reporting System (VAERS), the CDC Vaccine Schedule app, the complete ACIP recommendations, and the General Best Practices for Immunization and Outbreak Information [9]. The immunization schedule contains a large, easy-to-read, color-coded figure that includes each vaccine and the recommended schedule for children 18 years and younger. The catch-up schedule contains a figure that summarizes each vaccine's catch-up recommendations for children aged 4 months through 18 years. The medical indications section includes vaccines that might be indicated for children and adolescents aged 18 years and younger with certain indicated medical diagnoses. Specific medical indications include pregnancy, immunocompromised status (excluding human immunodeficiency virus [HIV] infection), HIV infection (further separated by total CD4 cell counts), kidney failure/end-stage renal disease/hemodialysis, heart and chronic lung disease, cerebrospinal fluid leaks and cochlear implants, asplenia and persistent complement component deficiencies, chronic liver disease, and diabetes. Lastly, there are 14 different notes that give further details for most vaccinations. Several modifications were made to the children and adolescent immunization schedule in February of 2019. These modifications included changes to the general schedule, influenza, hepatitis A, hepatitis B, and inactivated polio vaccine (IPV), and the addition of information regarding outbreaks [10].

General schedule changes

There were several changes to the general schedule. The changes to the cover page included a simpler design, shortening of the schedule title, the inclusion of basic instructions on how to use the schedule, and a list of routine vaccinations and combination vaccinations with their abbreviations and trade names. The cover page also added hyperlinks to the CDC Vaccine Schedules app, reference materials on vaccine-preventable disease surveillance, the VAERS, traveler's vaccines, and vaccine information sheets (VISs). The changes to the recommended vaccinations by medical condition and other indications include the differentiation between precautions for vaccination, delays in vaccination, and contraindications to vaccination. Precaution is defined as "vaccine might be indicated if benefit of protection outweighs risk of adverse reaction" [10]. Precautions are highlighted in orange. Delay in vaccination is defined as "vaccine that should not be given during pregnancy" [10]. Delays are highlighted in pink. Contraindicated or the use is not recommended is defined as "vaccine should not be administered because of risk factors for serious adverse reactions" [10]. Contraindications are highlighted in red [10]. These highlights make it easy to distinguish between the 3 precautions. The last pages of the schedule contain notes (previously termed footnotes) that have been rearranged in alphabetical order by vaccine name. These notes contain information regarding vaccine indications, dosing frequencies, dosing intervals, and other ACIP recommendations [10].

Influenza vaccine

There were numerous updates to the influenza vaccine in the 2019 schedule. A new statement is included that indicates any licensed influenza vaccine that is appropriate for the age and health status of the patient may be used. There are 2 separate preparations for influenza vaccine: inactivated influenza vaccine (IIV) and live attenuated influenza vaccine (LAIV). LAIV is now recommended in the 2018 to 2019 influenza season. IIV and LAIV are now separated into 2 rows on the immunization schedule. In addition, a list of exclusionary criteria is included for the use of LAIV. These exclusions or contraindications include children or adolescents who:

- Have immunocompromising conditions, including HIV
- Have anatomic or functional asplenia
- Are pregnant
- Have close contact with or are caregivers of severely immunocompromised persons in a protected environment
- Have received influenza antiviral medications in the previous 48 hours
- Have cerebrospinal fluid leak or a cochlear implant
- Are aged 2 to 4 years and have received a diagnosis of asthma or wheezing within the previous 12 months
- Are receiving medications containing aspirin or salicylate
- Have a history of severe allergic reaction to any component of the vaccine (except egg) or after a previous dose of any influenza vaccine [10]

Precautions for the LAIV include people with asthma who are 5 years or older, and people who have other underlying medical conditions such as chronic pulmonary, cardiovascular (except isolated hypertension), renal, hepatic, neurologic, hematologic, or metabolic disorders (including diabetes mellitus) [10].

Hepatitis A vaccine

Homelessness is now an indication for the hepatitis A (HepA) vaccine not only because of an increase in the number of outbreaks of hepatitis that have occurred in 11 states since 2016 but also because studies have shown homeless people to have 2 to 3 times higher risk of a HepA infection or disease [11]. HepA is also recommended for travelers 6 to 11 months of age and unvaccinated travelers aged 12 years or older because of these outbreaks. The HepA note was revised to include the use of the HepA-HepB combination vaccination, vaccination (Twinrix), in adolescents aged 18 years and older.

Hepatitis B vaccine

The HepB note has been updated to include information on HEPLISAV-B for use in people aged 18 years and older. The HEPLISAV-B vaccine was approved for use by the Food and Drug Administration (FDA) in November of 2017 [12].

Meningococcal serogroup B vaccine

The recommended vaccination by medical condition schedule has changed for the meningococcal serogroup B vaccine (MenB-4C or MenB-FHbp). The previous schedule listed this vaccine as recommended in pregnancy for persons with an additional risk factor for which the vaccine would be indicated. It has been changed to the orange, precaution, recommendation. There are a few smaller studies that do not indicate harm with these vaccinations; however, because of the lack of large studies completed on the safety of the MenB-4C or MenB-FHbp vaccines, it has been listed as a precaution in pregnancy [13].

Inactivated polio vaccine

For clarification purposes, a bullet has been added to the inactivated polio vaccine (IPV) note that indicates "4 or more doses of IPV can be administered before the 4th birthday when a combination vaccine containing IPV is used." An additional dose is also recommended after the fourth birthday and at least 6 months after the previous dose.

Tetanus, diphtheria, and pertussis vaccine

The Tdap row for adolescents aged 13 to 18 years has been split in half to reflect the catch-up schedule and use in pregnancy. Also, the Tdap note has been updated and clarified to include an additional dose of Tdap at the age of 11 to 12 years for children who inadvertently or as part of a catch-up series received a dose of diphtheria, tetanus and pertussis (DTaP) or Tdap at the age of 7 to 10 years. One dose of Tdap is recommended for each pregnancy. Also, a hyperlink to information on the use of Tdap or tetanus vaccine (Td) for tetanus prophylaxis in wound management has been added [14].

Outbreaks

The Additional Information section at the beginning of the notes page directs providers to their own state or local health departments for up-to-date information regarding vaccinations during an outbreak. Because this information was added to the notes, the information regarding additional doses of MMR and meningococcal (groups A, C, W-135, and Y) conjugate (MenACWY) or meningococcal serogroup B vaccines during outbreaks has been removed. The recent increase in outbreaks of measles, mumps, and meningitis have influenced the addition of this referral to state and local health departments [15–17].

2019 CHANGES TO THE ADULT IMMUNIZATION SCHEDULE

The adult immunization schedule was also updated in February of 2019 [18]. The adult schedule consists of a cover page, the recommended adult immunization schedule, recommendations by medical conditions and other indications, and notes. The cover page for the Recommended Adult Immunization Schedule for Ages 19 Years or Older, United States, 2019 includes general directions, notes on considerations for special populations, a listing of additional resources for health care providers, directions for reportable communicable diseases, and a table with abbreviations and trade names for each vaccine. The immunization schedule includes a table of age groups and recommended vaccines. The medical indications page includes vaccine recommendations based on medical conditions such as pregnancy, HIV infection, asplenia and complement deficiencies, end-stage renal disease and dialysis, heart or lung disease and alcoholism, chronic liver disease, diabetes, health care personnel, and men who have sex with men. The notes (previously footnotes) section contains more detailed information for each vaccine [18]. Changes to the 2019 adult immunization schedule included general schedule changes made to the cover page, figures, and notes as well as updates for 3 vaccination recommendations: influenza vaccine, HepA vaccine, and HepB vaccine [19].

General schedule changes

General schedule changes to the adult schedule were very similar to the changes noted earlier in the children and adolescent schedule. The cover page has a simplified design that includes directions on how to use the immunization schedule and a table of adult vaccines, their abbreviations, and trade names. It contains hyperlinks to the ACIP, the CDC, the ACOG, and the American Academy of Family Physicians (AAFP) Web sites. It contains a statement that encourages people to report suspected cases of reportable vaccine-preventable diseases to their local or state health department. It also has a hyperlink for vaccine injury claims to the Vaccine Injury Compensation Program, the CDC (including a telephone number), and the CDC Vaccine Schedule app. Other additional hyperlinks include the VAERS Web site, General Best Practice Guidelines for Immunization (including contraindications and precautions) Web site, VISs, Manual for the Surveillance of Vaccine-Preventable Diseases (including case identification and outbreak response), travel vaccine recommendations, and the Recommended Child and Adolescent Immunization Schedule for 2019. The recommended immunizations by medical conditions and other indications table has incorporated the precaution (orange), delay (pink), and contraindicated or use not recommended (red) highlights, which reflect the same definitions that are found in the child and adolescent schedule. The notes in the adult schedule have also been renamed (previously named Footnotes) and rearranged into alphabetical order by vaccine name. The notes include additional information on vaccine indications, dosing frequencies, dosing intervals, and other ACIP recommendations.

Influenza vaccine

Changes in the influenza vaccine are similar to the changes noted earlier in the children and adolescents schedule. Any licensed influenza vaccine that is appropriate for age and health status of the person may be used. Again, LAIV has been separated from IIV on the schedule. LAIV is an option for adults through the age of 49 years, except for those who:

- Have immunocompromising conditions, including HIV infection
- Have anatomic or functional asplenia
- Are pregnant
- Have close contact with or are caregivers of severely immunocompromised persons in a protected environment
- Have received influenza antiviral medication in the previous 48 hours
- Have a cerebrospinal fluid leak or a cochlear implant [19]

Hepatitis A vaccine

As mentioned earlier regarding the changes to the children and adolescent immunization schedule, homelessness is now an indication for the HepA vaccine. Two doses of HepA are recommended or 3 doses of the combination HepA-HepB (Twinrix) vaccine are recommended.

Hepatitis B vaccine

HEPLISAV-B has been added to the schedule and may be used routinely with 2 doses that are at least 4 weeks apart. As noted previously, HEPLISAV-B was approved by the FDA in November of 2017 [12].

SUMMARY

There were several key changes made to both the child and adolescent and adult immunization schedules in 2019. Key recommendation changes for the children and adolescents schedule included influenza, HepA, HepB, IPV, and Tdap vaccines. Key recommendation changes for the adult schedule included influenza, HepA, and HepB vaccines. The ACIP makes changes to the immunization schedules based on new scientific research and new available vaccinations. They publish these changes as needed to prevent disease and improve outcomes. Health care providers should know these changes and understand the rationale behind each change. Both immunization schedules can be found on the CDC Web site (https://www.cdc.gov/vaccines/schedules/) [3].

References

[1] Robinson CL, Romero JR, Kempe A, et al. Advisory committee on immunization practices recommended immunization schedule for children and adolescents aged 18 years or younger – United States, 2018. MMWR Morb Mortal Wkly Rep 2018;67:156–7.

[2] Centers for Disease Control and Prevention. Ten great public health achievements: United States, 2001-2010. Available at: https://www.cdc.gov/mmwr/preview/mmwrhtml/mm6019a5.htm. Accessed February 12, 2019.

[3] Centers for Disease Control and Prevention. Achievements in public health, 1990-1999: control of infectious diseases. Available at: https://www.cdc.gov/mmwr/preview/mmwrhtml/mm4829a1.htm. Accessed February 12, 2019.

[4] Centers for Disease Control and Prevention. Vaccines & immunizations. Available at: https://www.cdc.gov/vaccines/vac-gen/howvpd.htm. Accessed February 12, 2019.

[5] Centers for Disease Control and Prevention. Table 66. Vaccination coverage for selected diseases among children aged 19-35 months, by race, Hispanic origin, poverty level, and location of residence in metropolitan statistical area: United States, selected years 1998-2016. Available at: https://www.cdc.gov/nchs/data/hus/2017/066.pdf. Accessed February 12, 2019.

[6] Centers for Disease Control and Prevention. Table 67. Vaccination coverage for selected diseases among adolescents aged 13-17, by selected characteristics: United States years 2008-2016. Available at: https://www.cdc.gov/nchs/data/hus/2017/067.pdf. Accessed February 12, 2019.

[7] Centers for Disease Control and Prevention. Table 68. Influenza vaccination among adults aged 18 and over, by selected characteristics: United States, 1989-2016. Available at: https://www.cdc.gov/nchs/data/hus/2017/068.pdf. Accessed February 12, 2019.

[8] Centers for Disease Control and Prevention. Table 69. Pneumococcal vaccination among adults aged 18 and over, by selected characteristics: United States, selected years 1989-2016. Available at: https://www.cdc.gov/nchs/data/hus/2017/069.pdf. Accessed February 12, 2019.

[9] Centers for Disease Control and Prevention. Recommended immunization schedule for children and adolescents aged 18 years or younger, United States. 2019. Available at: https://www.cdc.gov/vaccines/schedules/downloads/child/0-18yrs-child-combined-schedule.pdf. Accessed February 12, 2019.

[10] Centers for Disease Control and Prevention. Immunization schedules: child immunization schedule changes for 2019. Available at: https://www.cdc.gov/vaccines/schedules/hcp/schedule-changes.html. Accessed February 12, 2019.

[11] American Academy of Family Physicians. ACIP recommends Hep A vaccine for homeless patients. Available at: https://www.aafp.org/news/health-of-the-public/20181031acipmeeting.html. Accessed February 12, 2019.

[12] The Department of Health and Human Services. The FDA approved the first new vaccine to prevent hepatitis B virus infection in 25 years. Available at: https://www.hhs.gov/hepatitis/blog/2017/11/29/fda-approves-new-hepatitis-b-vaccine/index.html. Accessed February 12, 2019.

[13] Makris MC, Polyzos KA, Mavros MN, et al. Safety of hepatitis B, pneumococcal polysaccharide and meningococcal polysaccharide vaccines in pregnancy. Available at: https://link-springer-com.proxy.lib.ohio-state.edu/article/10.2165%2F11595670-000000000-00000. Accessed February 12, 2019.

[14] Centers for Disease Control and Prevention. Prevention of pertussis, tetanus, and diphtheria with vaccines in the United States: recommendation of the Advisory Committee on Immunization Practices (ACIP). Available at: https://www.cdc.gov/mmwr/volumes/67/rr/rr6702a1.htm#. Accessed February 12, 2019.

[15] Centers for Disease Control and Prevention. Mumps cases and outbreaks. Available at: https://www.cdc.gov/mumps/outbreaks.html. Accessed February 12, 2019.

[16] Centers for Disease Control and Prevention. Measles cases and outbreaks. Available at: https://www.cdc.gov/measles/cases-outbreaks.html. Accessed February 12, 2019.

[17] Centers for Disease Control and Prevention. Manual for the surveillance of vaccine-preventable disease: chapter 8: meningococcal disease. Available at: https://www.cdc.gov/vaccines/pubs/surv-manual/chpt08-mening.html. Accessed February 12, 2019.

[18] Centers for Disease Control and Prevention. Recommended adult immunization schedule for ages 19 years or older, United States, 2019. Available at: https://www.cdc.gov/vaccines/schedules/downloads/adult/adult-combined-schedule.pdfhttps://www.cdc.gov/vaccines/schedules/downloads/adult/adult-combined-schedule.pdf. Accessed February 12, 2019.

[19] Centers for Disease Control and Prevention. Adult immunization schedule changes for 2019. Available at: https://www.cdc.gov/vaccines/schedules/hcp/schedule-changes.html. Accessed February 12, 2019.

Moving?

Make sure your subscription moves with you!

To notify us of your new address, find your **Clinics Account Number** (located on your mailing label above your name), and contact customer service at:

Email: **journalscustomerservice-usa@elsevier.com**

800-654-2452 (subscribers in the U.S. & Canada)
314-447-8871 (subscribers outside of the U.S. & Canada)

Fax number: **314-447-8029**

Elsevier Health Sciences Division
Subscription Customer Service
3251 Riverport Lane
Maryland Heights, MO 63043

*To ensure uninterrupted delivery of your subscription, please notify us at least 4 weeks in advance of move.

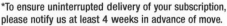

Printed and bound by CPI Group (UK) Ltd, Croydon, CR0 4YY

07/10/2024

01040501-0007